Cholesterol Cures

FEATURING

The Breakthrough Menu Plan
to *Slash* Cholesterol

Cholesterol Cures

By the Editors of
Rodale Health Books
Medical Advisor: William P. Castelli, MD

RODALE

Notice

This book is intended as a reference volume only, not as a medical manual. The information given here is designed to help you make informed decisions about your health. It is not intended as a substitute for any treatment that may have been prescribed by your doctor. If you suspect that you have a medical problem, we urge you to seek competent medical care.

Mention of specific companies, organizations, or authorities in this book does not imply endorsement by the publisher, nor does mention of specific companies, organizations, or authorities imply their endorsement of this book.

Internet addresses and telephone numbers in this book were accurate at the time it went to press.

Rodale books may be purchased for business or promotional use or for special sales. For information, please write to: Special Markets Department, Rodale Inc., 733 Third Avenue, New York, NY 10017.

Printed in the United States of America

Rodale Inc. makes every effort to use acid-free ∞, recycled paper ♻

Book design by Christopher Rhoads

Library of Congress Cataloging-in-Publication Data

Cholesterol cures : featuring the breakthrough menu plan to slash cholesterol / by the editors of Rodale Health Books. — Rev. and updated ed.
    p.   cm.
Includes index.
ISBN-13 978-1-59486-735-4 paperback
ISBN-10 1-59486-735-6 paperback
1. Low-cholesterol diet—Popular works.   2. Hypocholesteremia—Diet therapy—Popular works.   3. Cholesterol—Popular works.   I. Rodale Health Books.
RM237.75.T78   2007
613.2'84—dc22   2007037835

Distributed to the trade by Holtzbrinck Publishers
    10   9   paperback

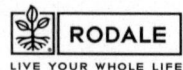

RODALE
LIVE YOUR WHOLE LIFE™

We inspire and enable people to improve their lives and the world around them
For more of our products visit **rodalestore.com** or call 800-848-4735

CONTENTS

PART ONE

Your Cholesterol-Reducing Action Plan

PART TWO

The Breakthrough Menu Plan

PART THREE

The 500-Food Fat and Cholesterol Counter

In 1948, the town of Framingham, Massachusetts, gave the world a great gift. Half of its residents allowed doctors to study them—and, in the decades that followed, their children, grandchildren, and great-grandchildren—to help the medical community unravel the mysteries of heart attack and stroke. For nearly 60 years, this study—known as the Framingham Heart Study—has been used to reveal the three biggest risk factors of heart disease: high levels of LDL cholesterol (the bad stuff; more about LDL in the following pages), high blood pressure, and smoking. The Big Three are followed closely by overweight, lack of exercise, diabetes, and stress.

Some of you might be wondering, "Aren't some people genetically predisposed to high cholesterol?" The answer is yes. But as the risk factors above show, we have to take some responsibility for having high cholesterol. After all, about 4 billion of the 5.7 billion people on the planet don't have high cholesterol. The average cholesterol level in central China, for example, is 125 milligrams/deciliter (mg/dl). The Masai people of Africa have cholesterol levels averaging 135 mg/dl. And in the less urban sections of Latin America, cholesterol levels hover under 150 mg/dl.

Fortunately, we can undo the harm caused by high-fat diets, inactivity, and other harmful factors. That's where this book comes in. It focuses on cholesterol cures—that is, simple things that virtually anyone can do to lower his or her blood cholesterol. Most of these cures focus on the foods we eat (or don't eat) and the lifestyle choices we make. This book also provides scores of no-cholesterol and low-fat menus and recipes that can help you start *now* to lower your cholesterol—to help you reap the health benefits right away.

But be advised: There's no such thing as a magic bullet. Choosing to take antioxidant supplements, for example, or to eat more garlic while continuing to eat a high-fat diet is unlikely to affect your cholesterol for the better. And use your common sense: Consider these cures as an adjunct to a doctor's care, particularly if your cholesterol is over 200 mg/dl.

For years, the American Heart Association; the National Cholesterol Education Program of the National Heart, Lung, and Blood Institute (part of the

National Institutes of Health in Bethesda, Maryland); and other health organizations have run huge public service campaigns to alert the public to the risk factors that can lead to heart disease. So many of us know what we have to do to take care of our hearts. But knowledge is useless if it's not paired with action.

I encourage you to mount your own personal campaign. To do so is to validate one of the foremost conclusions of the Framingham Heart Study: that the promise—and the privilege—of good health lies in our own hands.

—William P. Castelli, MD
Cardiologist at the Heart Center of MetroWest in Framingham, Massachusetts, and former director of the Framingham Heart Study

Getting to Know the "Good" and the "Bad"

With all the bad press it receives, you might be surprised to learn that cholesterol isn't actually bad for you.

Quite the contrary, cholesterol—like sweat, mucus, and many other unsavory substances produced by the body—is vital to your health and well-being. It's found in every cell, and the fatlike substance is a vital building block in the formation of some hormones.

The problem is that your body produces all the cholesterol it needs on its own. And—as cholesterol-lowering medication commercials are more than willing to tell us—the extra comes from two sources: your family and your diet. Regardless of what is causing it, high blood cholesterol is a cause for major concern: It sets the stage for a host of debilitating health conditions, including arteriosclerosis (hardening of the arteries), heart attack, and stroke. The other frightening aspect of high cholesterol is that many of the people who have it don't even know it. High cholesterol exhibits no signs or symptoms until it progresses into a more serious condition, so the only way to know if you have it is to get tested (more on this later).

When you consider how common high cholesterol is, the numbers are staggering: More than 105 million American adults have blood cholesterol levels above 200 milligrams/deciliter (mg/dl), and more than 36 million of those have levels above 240 mg/dl. (According to the American Heart Association, levels above 200 mg/dl put people at borderline-high risk, while levels above 240 mg/dl are designated high risk.) Moreover, high cholesterol doesn't seem to discriminate: Based on the American Heart Association's most recent statistics, population groups across the board—white, black, Hispanic; men and women—all have similarly high cholesterol numbers. It truly is a national epidemic in its scale.

That's the bad news. The good news is that few, if any, medical conditions are more preventable through lifestyle changes than high blood cholesterol.

This is one condition where diet doesn't play a *supporting* role—it's your primary means of defense.

And there's more good news: Taking control of your cholesterol levels can also prevent or reduce other related heart problems. "There are solid studies showing that watching your diet, exercising regularly, and reducing your stress level can slow or even reverse atherosclerosis," says Marianne Legato, MD, associate professor of clinical medicine at Columbia University College of Physicians and Surgeons in New York City.

If your cholesterol is within acceptable limits, this book can help you keep it there. Should it be off the charts, these doctor-recommended hints, tips, and suggestions can help you knock it back, perhaps averting the need for expensive medication—or even surgery.

Even if you've already been diagnosed with heart disease, there's reason for hope. Research shows that people with severe heart disease can turn their health around. One study, the Multicenter Lifestyle Demonstration Project, led by Dean Ornish, MD, president and director of the Preventive Medicine Research Institute in Sausalito, California, was designed to determine the effectiveness and cost savings of a healthier lifestyle program. It showed that people who were eligible for bypass surgery or angioplasty were able to avoid it for at least 3 years by making lifestyle changes recommended in hospital programs that followed Dr. Ornish's guidelines.

A previous study, the Lifestyle Heart Trial, also led by Dr. Ornish, concluded that people with heart disease can often stop, or even reverse, their conditions with lifestyle changes alone. Most likely, you can do it, too.

Six Reasons to Wage a Plaque Attack

To fire up your resolve, here's a list of the most significant benefits of reducing your cholesterol.

You can slow or even reverse the progression of atherosclerosis. It's not cholesterol alone that leads to heart disease. Rather, too much cholesterol in the blood can lead to fatty deposits of plaque building up on the walls of the coronary arteries, the vessels that supply oxygen-rich blood to the heart. This condition is known as atherosclerosis. If left untreated, these blockages can choke off the heart's supply of blood, leading to chest pain (angina), heart attack, or even death.

Lowering your cholesterol can reduce your chances of atherosclerosis and coronary heart disease. One landmark study of 3,806 men with high choles-terol, the Lipid Research Clinics Coronary Primary Prevention Trial, found that those whose cholesterol levels dropped by 13 to 20 percent also experi-enced a reduction in their chances of developing coronary heart disease (19 percent) and their risk of having a heart attack (24 percent).

You can reduce or eliminate your reliance on cholesterol-lowering medication. Cholesterol-lowering medications undoubtedly play a role in the treatment of high blood cholesterol, particularly among people who blame their high cholesterol on their family history, as well among those with extremely high cholesterol. The most commonly prescribed cholesterol-lowering drugs are the statins, which include atorvastatin (Lipitor) and simva-statin (Zocor), among many others. Other families of cholesterol-lowering drugs include bile-acid-binding resins (Prevalite, Questran), cholesterol absorption inhibitors (Zetia), and a combination statin/inhibitor (Vytorin).

Though these drugs are helpful and necessary for many with high choles-terol, "drugs are the second line of defense," says John McDougall, MD, founder of the McDougall Program and McDougall Health Clinic in Santa Rosa, California (www.DrMcDougall.com). "Diet and lifestyle changes are the foundation for recovering from coronary heart disease."

You can reduce your risk of stroke. In most cases, heart attack and stroke have virtually identical causes: instead of restricted blood flow to the heart, a stroke occurs because of restricted blood flow to the brain. So it

Men: Lower Your Cholesterol, Improve Your Love Life?

Men with high total cholesterol and low levels of good HDL cholesterol may be prime candidates for erectile difficulty, several studies show.

In one study, researchers gave a group of 3,371 men physical exams, includ-ing cholesterol tests. Each man visited the clinic twice, with an average of 22 months between visits.

In that time, 71 men developed difficulty achieving or maintaining erections. Men with total cholesterol levels above 240 milligrams/deciliter (mg/dl) were 83 percent more likely to experience the problem than men whose total cho-lesterol was below 180 mg/dl. Also, men whose HDL exceeded 60 mg/dl were 70 percent less likely to have difficulty than men whose HDL was below 30 mg/dl. Atherosclerosis may cause the problem by reducing blood flow to the penis, the researchers speculated.

Another study, which examined the various causes of erectile difficulty in Massachusetts men, found that the men's risk rose as their HDL levels dipped.

makes sense that reducing your cholesterol can help prevent stroke just as it prevents a heart attack.

But cholesterol may play another role in strokes as well. One study found that elevated cholesterol can produce abnormal amounts of a chemical that can cause spasms in the carotid artery in the neck, which supplies blood to the brain. If these spasms interrupt blood flow, they could cause a mini-stroke, or transient ischemic attack.

If you have diabetes, you can prevent it from leading to other problems. Keeping your cholesterol under control can prove doubly important if you have diabetes. That's because some research suggests that both women and men with diabetes have about twice the coronary heart disease risk of the general population and, if they've had a coronary event, are twice as

---

Will HRT Help? It Depends

Before they reach menopause, women have significantly lower rates of coronary heart disease than men of the same ages. Why? In a word: estrogen. This female sex hormone appears to raise women's stores of heart-healthy HDL cholesterol. "Women tend to have higher HDL than men, which may be why they have less heart disease than men—at least in their premenopausal years," says Peter Wood, DSc, PhD, professor emeritus of medicine at Stanford University School of Medicine.

After the onset of menopause, a woman's levels of total and LDL cholesterol rise and her HDL wanes, most likely due to a dwindling supply of estrogen. Eventually, postmenopausal women find that their risk of heart disease and heart attack catches up to that of men the same age. Despite this, women can protect themselves in the same ways that men do: by quitting smoking, losing weight, eating a healthy diet, and getting regular exercise.

For many women and their doctors, hormone replacement therapy (HRT, comprised of estrogen or estrogen and progesterone) has been the treatment of choice for the changes typically associated with menopause, from temporary discomforts like hot flashes to long-term consequences like decreasing bone density. HRT was once considered beneficial to women's heart health, but new evidence suggests that for some women, the opposite may be true. One large study suggested that it seems to increase the risk of death in women who already have heart disease when they begin treatment. The evidence is strong enough that most health experts now recommend avoiding hormone replacement therapy for women at high risk of developing heart disease.

Your best bet? "Discuss HRT with your doctor before menopause so that you'll have a plan in place once it happens," advises Debra Judelson, MD, medical director of the Women's Heart Institute at the Cardiovascular Medical Group in Los Angeles.

likely to suffer repeat problems, such as heart attacks, angina, and the need for bypass surgery. People with diabetes also tend to have high levels of tri-glycerides, another blood fat implicated in coronary heart disease. If you have diabetes, lowering your cholesterol and controlling other risk factors such as high blood pressure and obesity can cut your chances of developing diabetes-related heart and blood vessel problems.

You can live longer. The renowned Framingham Heart Study, which tracked the health of the residents of Framingham, Massachusetts, for more than 4 decades, has shown that the lower cholesterol levels fall, the lower the chance of heart attack and sudden death.

You can enhance your quality of life. Taking charge of elevated cho-lesterol now could mean the difference between a future of shuttling to and from the doctor's office (or the hospital) and enjoying a full, happy, healthy life.

Getting to Know Cholesterol

Cholesterol is a soft, waxy substance found in every human cell, in blood, and in food. The kind found in food is called dietary cholesterol. Only animal-based foods such as meat and dairy products contain dietary cholesterol; it's not found in plant-based foods such as fruits, vegetables, beans, and grains.

As established earlier, cholesterol isn't as evil as you might think. Your liver, for example, uses cholesterol to make bile acids, which help you digest food. In fact, one of the two major types of cholesterol in the body can actu-ally *improve* your health.

More Than One Kind of Blood Fat Is Involved

You've probably heard your doctor talk about "good" cholesterol and "bad" cholesterol. Cholesterol doesn't dissolve in blood, so it can't get to where the body needs it on its own. It has to hitch a ride on special carriers called lipoproteins. The lipoproteins that are considered good are known as high-density lipoproteins, or HDL. They're called high-density because they're mostly protein.

The other major lipoprotein, the "bad" kind, is known as low-density lipoprotein, or LDL. And as you probably guessed, LDL is packed with cho-lesterol.

Though similar in name, LDL and HDL actually do two dramatically different things as they traverse the bloodstream.

If there's too much LDL in your blood, it gets deposited on the walls of your arteries as fatty clumps. If these clumps break free, they can cause the blood to clot. A clot that cuts off the flow of blood to the heart can cause a heart attack; a clot that blocks blood flow to the brain can trigger a stroke. HDL, on the other hand, is a cardiovascular hero. It patrols your arteries, hauling cholesterol away from them and carrying it to the liver for dumping.

Now, like most things in life, these distinctions make your cholesterol test (which, by the way, you should get at least every 5 years, and more often if your doctor says you should) a little more complicated. But in this case, the complication is worth it, as it can give you a clear picture of exactly where your cholesterol levels should be.

How High Is High?

Some people can rattle off their cholesterol levels as quickly as their Social Security numbers. But if you require some translation, consult these guidelines, designated by the National Cholesterol Education Program of the National Institutes of Health and updated in 2004. (All readings are in milligrams/deciliter.)

Total Cholesterol

Desirable	Less than 200
Borderline high	200 to 239
High	240 or above

LDL Cholesterol

Optimal for people at very high risk of heart disease	Less than 70
Optimal for people at risk of heart disease	Less than 100
Near optimal	100 to 129
Borderline high	130 to 159
High	160 to 189
Very high	190 or above

HDL Cholesterol

Poor	Less than 40
Better	40 to 59
Best	60 or above

As mentioned before, you want your total cholesterol level to be below 200 mg/dl. In addition to this, though, your level of LDL cholesterol is quite important. It breaks down as shown in "How High Is High?" As you can see, that's quite a range of LDL levels to strive for.

If you've had a heart attack or have diabetes, that places you firmly in the "very high risk" category. Two or more of the following factors might also place you in the "very high risk" group: if you smoke, have high blood pressure, have low HDL cholesterol, have a family history of heart disease, or are a man over age 45 or a woman over 55.

Then there is your HDL cholesterol level, which—you may have guessed—you actually *want* to be higher. Here, anything below 40 mg/dl is considered poor, 40 to 59 mg/dl is considered good, and 60 mg/dl and above is the best.

Whenever you have a cholesterol test, the lab will also measure your triglyceride level, since many people with high triglycerides have high LDL or low HDL levels. Triglyceride levels of less than 150 mg/dl are considered desirable.

Additionally, it's a good idea to know your level of lipoprotein(a), or LP(a). LP(a) is a chunk of cholesterol coated with protein, and it's found only in the blood of hedgehogs, certain monkeys—and humans.

Researchers at Oxford University in England found that among people who had heart disease or who had survived a heart attack, those with the highest levels of LP(a) also had a 70 percent greater risk of having a heart attack over a 10-year period than those with the lowest levels. Levels starting at 30 mg/dl seem to raise risk. The Framingham Heart Study found that having levels of about 30 mg/dl doubled the risk of heart attack in 3,000 women. So an LP(a) test is something to consider if you are female or have heart disease or a family history of premature coronary artery disease or stroke.

Size Matters

In the last decade, scientists have developed an even more sophisticated understanding of HDL and LDL cholesterol. As it turns out, it's not just the type of cholesterol that matters, it's also the size.

It seems that for both LDL and HDL, larger lipoproteins are preferable. Larger LDL particles are less likely to embed themselves in the walls of your arteries and lead to atherosclerosis and heart disease, for example. And larger particles of HDL are more likely to grab onto harmful particles and shuttle them out of the body.

Though more research is needed, it seems that some foods, such as eggs, may not be as risky as they were previously thought to be, as they prompt the body to manufacture larger lipoproteins, rather than smaller ones. Stay tuned for more studies about the size of cholesterol lipoproteins in the near future.

Updated Government Cholesterol Guidelines Call for More Attention to Diet and Lifestyle

Lifestyle changes—the clinician's shorthand for healthy eating, regular exercise, and weight control—are the first line of defense against high cholesterol and heart disease.

That's the word from the National Cholesterol Education Program's Adult Treatment Panel III (ATP III) report. (The National Cholesterol Education Program is an initiative of the National Heart, Lung, and Blood Institute, part of the National Institutes of Health.) First issued in 2001, the recommendations of the ATP III report were updated slightly in 2004, after the National Cholesterol Education Program reviewed the results of five major clinical trials that tested the ATP III guidelines. Here are the recommendations for preventing and treating high cholesterol that came from the culmination of these two reports:

- Treat high cholesterol more aggressively in people with type 2 diabetes. They're at particularly high risk of dying from a heart attack.

- Set a new level at which low HDL cholesterol becomes a risk factor for heart disease. Reflecting recent findings about the strong link between low HDL and heart disease, low HDL is now defined as being below 40 milligrams/deciliter (mg/dl), up from 35 mg/dl.

- Set a new optimal level of LDL cholesterol for people at very high risk of heart disease. Those include people who have diabetes, have previously had a heart attack, or exhibit two or more risk factors, such as smoking, low HDL cholesterol, high blood pressure, a family history of heart disease, or being a man over 45 or a woman over 55. This new level is 70 mg/dl, down from 100 mg/dl.

- Advocate a more in-depth initial test for high cholesterol. The first test should be a complete lipoprotein profile—including total, HDL, and LDL cholesterol and triglyceride levels—rather than just total and HDL cholesterol levels.

What's Your Ratio?

Most likely, you're familiar with your total cholesterol, which actually is the sum of your HDL and LDL values and those of other blood fats. To see if your blood fats fall within a desirable range, your doctor will determine your cholesterol ratio—that is, your total cholesterol divided by your HDL number.

The theory is that combining the levels into one number will give you an overall look at your individual heart disease risk. Experts agree that the ideal

The National Institutes of Health has developed an online calculator to help men and women determine their risk for heart attack over the next 10 years. To find this tool, go to their Web site at http://rover.nhlbi.nih.gov/guidelines/cholesterol and click on "10-Year Risk Calculator for Patients."

Lifestyle changes alone can lower cholesterol levels in some folks with elevated cholesterol. But more beans, greens, and brisk walks can also benefit the 13 million men and women who take cholesterol-lowering drugs, according to the authors of the report.

Compared with the previous ATP report, issued in 1993, ATP III places more emphasis on "therapeutic lifestyle changes," or TLC—rather than medication—as the first treatment for elevated cholesterol and particularly for "bad" LDL cholesterol, which is a major cause of coronary heart disease.

There are four components of TLC.

- To reduce intake of saturated fat—the artery-clogging fat found in foods like bacon, butter, and full-fat cheese—to less than 7 percent of total daily calories and to limit intake of dietary cholesterol to no more than 200 milligrams a day.

- To get 10 to 25 grams (2 to 5 teaspoons) per day of soluble fiber, found in foods such as cereal grains, beans, fruits, and vegetables. It also encourages the use of foods that contain sterols and stanols. These plant substances are found in some types of spreads and salad dressings, such as Benecol and Take Control.

- To get at least 30 minutes of physical activity a day.

- To lose weight.

The information and advice that are given in this book have been updated and revised to help you achieve all of those heart-healthy diet and lifestyle goals.

ratio is 3.5 to 1 or lower, although many feel that it's even more important to pay attention to the individual values, since levels of both LDL and HDL play a role in predicting heart health.

Let's say you learn that your total cholesterol is 250 mg/dl and your HDL is 50 mg/dl (above the desired minimum of 40 mg/dl). Dividing your total cholesterol (250) by your HDL (50) gives you a ratio of 5 to 1. But cutting your total cholesterol to 200 mg/dl (the new desired maximum) while holding your HDL at 50 mg/dl will shrink your ratio to a more desirable 4 to 1. In fact, doctors participating in the Physicians' Health Study—an ongoing study of more than 22,000 American doctors conducted at Harvard Medical School and Brigham and Women's Hospital in Boston—found that cutting just one unit from their ratios of total to HDL cholesterol slashed their heart attack risk by 53 percent!

Five Proven Ways to Lower Your Cholesterol

There are dozens of options, both major and minor, for lowering your cholesterol. To help you focus and prioritize your choices, try the following simple five-step approach.

1. Choose your fats wisely. Most people now get about 37 percent of total calories from fat, down from 42 percent in the 1960s. This is great news, since consuming too much fat, particularly saturated fat, has been linked to an increased risk of coronary heart disease. But we still have a way to go: The American Heart Association recommends getting no more than 30 percent of calories from fat. Other experts suggest 25 percent or even less.

   While cutting back on saturated fat is an excellent move, it's actually a better idea to eat more monounsaturated fat—found in olive and canola oils, most nuts (almonds, walnuts, peanuts and peanut butter, and pecans), and avocados—than to eliminate all fat. In one study, a diet high in monounsaturated fat lowered triglycerides in overweight men.

2. Get serious about losing weight. People who follow low-fat, low-cholesterol diets and lose excess weight tend to have an easier time reducing their levels of total and LDL cholesterol than people who don't drop the extra pounds. Being overweight seems to disrupt the normal metabolism of fats, which means that even if you eat less fat (a common first step in trying to clobber cholesterol), you won't get the biggest heart benefits unless you lose weight as well.

   One study of 150 overweight people concluded that those who lose just 10 to 15 percent of excess body weight—and keep it off—may afford themselves long-term protection from coronary heart disease.

   Dropping extra pounds may also boost HDL cholesterol. In a study of

A Cornucopia of Natural Cholesterol "Prescriptions"

Before you proceed to the cholesterol-busting natural remedies contained within the pages of this book, here's one caveat: If your doctor determines that you need medication to reduce your cholesterol levels, it's best to listen. Great strides have been made in cholesterol medication over the last decade, and a number of options are available to keep cholesterol in check.

At the same time, it's not unrealistic to reduce or even end your dependence on medication through strict adherence to a healthy diet, an exercise regimen, and some of the remedies found within this book. After all, since diet is the number one reason Americans have problems with cholesterol to begin with, it would stand to reason that diet would also be part of the solution.

2,400 people, women experienced a 2 percent increase in LDL and a 2 percent drop in HDL for every 5 pounds they gained.

Research from the landmark Framingham Heart Study shows that weight loss helps your health in other ways. Taking off 1 to 2 pounds a year—and maintaining the loss—may cut your risk of high blood pressure by 25 percent and your risk of diabetes by 35 percent.

3. Step up your efforts to exercise. Researchers at Stanford University found that people who teamed exercise with a low-fat diet doubled their LDL reduction. They participated in 30 minutes of moderate exercise at least three times a week. Accumulating 45 to 60 minutes of moderate-intensity activity at least 5 days a week also helps you lose weight.

4. If you smoke, quit once and for all. Smoking can lead to atherosclerosis and can reduce HDL by as much as 15 percent. Within 2 years after you quit, however, your risk of heart disease is about the same as that of someone who never smoked, says Lori Mosca, MD, PhD, director of preventive cardiology at New York–Presbyterian Hospital and associate professor of medicine at Columbia University in New York. So quitting can significantly improve your cholesterol profile.

"Quitting smoking can reverse the negative effect on HDL in just 60 days," explains Robert Rosenson, MD, director of the Preventive Cardiology Center at the University of Michigan Medical Center in Ann Arbor.

5. Reduce your stress levels. Chronic stress may raise levels of homocysteine, an amino acid that's been linked to increased heart disease risk in men and women. So, keeping cool may help keep the lid on your cholesterol.

In the chapters that follow, you will learn about practical, expert-recommended strategies that can help you wallop high cholesterol without the use of prescription drugs. Some of these tactics may sound familiar; others are on the cutting edge of medical research. Provided that your physician gives you the green light, you can add virtually all of these strategies to your daily routine with a minimum of time, money, and effort.

Along the way, you'll gain a wealth of practical information that can help you achieve your ultimate goal—a heart-healthy cholesterol level. You will discover:

• How olives, peanut butter, avocados, and other indulgences can help boost your good cholesterol and lower your bad cholesterol

• Why folks in certain parts of the world seem to enjoy better heart health than we do, and why some experts continue to steer us toward the kinds of foods favored in Mediterranean diets

• Ongoing research that suggests certain vitamins and minerals may help reduce cholesterol and protect against coronary heart disease

• Tips from chefs who've mastered the art of reducing fat and cholesterol in their recipes without reducing flavor

• A comprehensive table of the total and saturated fat contents of 500 common foods

As a bonus, we've devised a time-tested, cholesterol-busting menu plan designed to drop your total cholesterol 30 points in 30 days while improving your HDL reading. You'll find this plan—created and reviewed by nutritionists—as delicious as it is effective.

Think of this plan as your own personal cholesterol-reduction tool. The sooner you put it to work, the sooner you'll reap your reward: a strong, healthy heart primed to provide years of vibrant living.

PART ONE

Your Cholesterol-Reducing Action Plan

Alcohol

Moderation Is the Key

When it comes to your heart health, few things have generated mixed messages quite like alcohol.

A big reason for this is the results of a number of studies over the last decade. These have shown that alcohol has a slew of heart-protective properties, including raising levels of "good" HDL cholesterol, lowering blood pressure, inhibiting the creation of blood clots, and just overall reducing the risk of coronary heart disease.

This, not surprisingly, got a number of people quite excited about the prospects. (Drinking protects the heart? All right!) But that excitement should be tempered somewhat. Experts unanimously agree that these studies do not give people a green light to go on a bender.

Alcohol presents a classic catch-22 for health professionals. Sure, it might protect the heart somewhat, but are the risks worth the benefit? The downside of alcohol is that it introduces a lot of dangers. If you or your family has been touched by alcoholism, you know how scary it can be. And with alcohol abuse, the risks to health are great: They include cancer, heart attack, stroke, depression, and cirrhosis of the liver, among many others.

The sage advice here, as with most things in life, is that moderation is the key. And in this case, health experts define moderation as no more than two drinks a day if you're a male under 65, and no more than one drink a day if you're a male over 65 or a female.

Also, if you're not a drinker, don't start just because it might help your heart. There are a number of other heart-protective strategies at your fingertips, and the risks of drinking are just too great. Whether or not you imbibe, read on to learn about the benefits and risks of alcohol.

The Benefits of Limited Consumption

Two studies looked at the relationship between drinking habits and cholesterol and triglyceride levels in women. One study, conducted in Finland, first tracked 274 healthy, middle-aged women with varied drinking habits and then followed up with an analysis of alcoholic women while they abstained from drinking. Among the study participants, total and HDL cholesterol levels improved, but LDL levels did not. The effect was most noticeable in women who reported drinking between ⅔ ounce and almost 1½ ounces of alcohol a day—about the equivalent of a small glass of wine, half a can of beer, or a mixed drink. When they drank more than 1½ ounces, all cholesterol values increased except for LDL. When the women then abstained for 2 weeks, their HDL dropped and their LDL cholesterol increased.

Other researchers examined the effect of slightly higher alcohol consumption on cardiovascular risk factors in women so they could compare the effect to that previously observed in men. In this study, the women—who were either postmenopausal or premenopausal and taking oral contraceptives—drank three glasses of either red wine or grape juice with dinner every day for 3 weeks. After 3 weeks, the researchers took blood samples 1 hour before dinner and then at 2- or 4-hour intervals for up to 19 hours after dinner. In both premenopausal and postmenopausal women, levels of both triglycerides and very low density lipoprotein (VLDL, an even more harmful type of LDL) peaked 3 hours after a dinner with wine. In addition, after drinking wine, the premenopausal women had a 12 percent increase in overall HDL cholesterol levels, and the postmenopausal women's LDL cholesterol levels decreased by the same amount, when compared with grape juice consumption. The response of postmenopausal women to alcohol resembled the response found in earlier studies in men.

According to data from the second National Health and Nutrition Examination Survey, average levels of HDL cholesterol were higher among drinkers than among abstainers, no matter what their age, gender, or race. Also, as alcohol consumption increased, so did HDL levels—an average increase of 5.1 milligrams/deciliter for daily or weekly use. (This study suggests, however, reducing your risk of coronary heart disease by means other than alcohol consumption.)

For 7 years, the Multiple Risk Factor Intervention Trial followed a subgroup consisting of 11,688 middle-aged men who were at high risk for heart disease. During that time, those who consumed about two drinks per day (with each drink equal to 4 ounces of wine, 12 ounces of beer, or 1½ ounces of 80-proof spirits) had higher HDL levels than nondrinkers. This alcohol intake seemed largely responsible for a 22 percent reduced chance of death from heart disease, researchers said.

At Kaiser Permanente Medical Center in Oakland, California, researchers tracked the alcohol consumption patterns of nearly 129,000 people. Those who had one to two drinks a day were 30 percent less likely to die from coronary heart disease than those who did not drink. But people who had six or more drinks a day had a 60 percent greater risk of death from noncardiovascular causes than nondrinkers.

In another study at Johns Hopkins University in Baltimore, researchers had 56 men with low levels of HDL either drink one beer a day or abstain from alcohol. After 2 months, there were no differences in HDL levels between the two groups. But the beer drinkers experienced a 10 percent increase in apolipoprotein A-1, the major protein component of HDL. This protein is believed to help extract cholesterol from the cells and move it to the liver for excretion. Alcohol also makes blood platelets less sticky, which cuts the risk of clot formation and reduces the risk of heart attack, and raises blood levels of an enzyme called tissue-type plasminogen activator, or tPA, which helps keep blood clots from forming.

Researchers at Harvard University and Brigham and Women's Hospital in Boston measured blood levels of tPA in 631 male doctors. These doctors—participants in the Physicians' Health Study, a study of 22,000 American doctors—gave blood samples and reported on their drinking habits. Researchers found that tPA levels rose with drinking frequency. The doctors who consumed two or more drinks a day had 35 percent higher levels of tPA than doctors who rarely or never drank. What's more, the doctors who drank more had significantly higher levels of HDL cholesterol than the doctors who didn't.

Does What You Drink Matter?

Other studies have looked at the issue of which drinks seem to offer the most heart-protective benefits. The results have been mixed, with a few studies indicating that some drinks (such as red wine and dark beer) are more protective, while other studies seem to indicate that the protective benefits are pretty consistent no matter what you drink.

A lot of the research in this area has been conducted by John D. Folts, PhD, director of the University of Wisconsin Coronary Artery Thrombosis Research and Prevention Lab at the University of Wisconsin Hospital and Clinics in Madison. According to Dr. Folts's research, what sets red wine and dark beer apart from other alcoholic beverages are their high levels of flavonoids, chemical compounds found in fruits, vegetables, and certain beverages. In red wine and beer, the flavonoids appear to make blood-clotting cells less sticky, so they are less likely to adhere to arterial walls.

Because Dr. Folts's studies on red wine and beer were conducted with laboratory animals, some skeptics believe human studies are needed to show whether or not flavonoids really add any value to the heart-protective benefits of alcoholic beverages. But in the meantime, Dr. Folts adds that you can get the most benefit from dark beer and red wine by imbibing with meals. This will help fight the oxidative stress that comes from metabolizing food, he says. Oxidative stress causes the wear and tear on the heart and arteries.

Not a Magic Bullet

If you think that simply hoisting a beer stein or sipping your favorite Bordeaux will be all that you need to do to improve your cholesterol level, think again. "Two glasses of wine a day will have a modest effect on your HDL, and even that modest effect is beneficial," says William P. Castelli, MD, a cardiologist at the Heart Center of MetroWest in Framingham, Massachusetts, and former director of the Framingham Heart Study. "But if you're looking for a magic bullet, this isn't it."

Further, overimbibing to benefit your cholesterol level is risky, say experts. "Alcohol is like coffee—it has some theoretical benefits and some potential risks," says Neal Barnard, MD, president of the Physicians Committee for Responsible Medicine in Washington, D.C.

Considering the great risks that can stem from alcohol abuse, most of the health experts in this chapter offer a simple solution. If you're concerned about your heart health, always speak with your doctor before choosing alcohol as a possible remedy. Your doctor can help you weigh the risks and benefits, and provide sound advice on how it should be consumed responsibly.

See also Flavonoids, Grape Juice, Grape Seed Extract, Red Wine

Antioxidants

The Plaque-Attacking Cardio-Nutrients

Antioxidants get a lot of good press these days, and there are a lot of good reasons why. But most sources don't tell you what antioxidants are and how they can help.

In order to understand the arterial heroes that are antioxidants, you first need to understand their archenemies, free radicals. Your body is under attack every day from free radicals. These are unstable oxygen molecules that enter the body through sources such as cigarette smoke, pollution, and even vigorous exercise. Once inside, they try to cure their instability by stealing electrons from a number of parts of your body, including the arterial walls. The damage caused by the free radicals in the arteries makes it easy for cholesterol to deposit itself, contributing to atherosclerosis and heart disease.

This is where our heroes, antioxidants, step in. When you eat fruits, vegetables, and other antioxidant-rich foods, these protective compounds enter the bloodstream and put themselves directly between the free radicals and your body's healthy molecules. By giving up their own electrons to the free radicals as a sacrifice, they keep your body out of harm's way.

Putting Antioxidants In

Now that you know what they are, you can understand how important it is to get more antioxidants into your body. And the best way to do that is to eat more fruits and vegetables. These heart-healthy superstars are packed with the "big three" antioxidants: vitamins C and E and beta-carotene, which converts to vitamin A in the body. They also are brimming with flavonoids, antioxidant compounds that have gained a great deal of attention in the research community lately.

In years past, some studies leaned toward taking supplements of antioxidants to gain even more of their heart-protective properties. But recent research has raised some doubts about the effectiveness of supplementation.

Vitamin C, in particular, has not produced dramatic benefits when taken in supplement form. And vitamin E has been shown to be dangerous and to raise the risk of death when taken in amounts greater than 200 IU a day. Beta-carotene supplementation also can be dangerous, particularly to smokers. "One thing we learned in two large studies about beta-carotene is that in smokers, there was actually a worse outcome in terms of cancer, death, and cardiovascular disease," says Howard N. Hodis, MD, director of the atherosclerosis research unit at the University of Southern California School of Medicine in Los Angeles. "So it appears that in concert with smoking, beta-carotene becomes an even worse actor. Certainly smokers should not be taking beta-carotene."

For these reasons, the most recent advice from the American Heart Association is to get your antioxidants by eating a plentiful array of fruits and vegetables. Read on to learn more about the pros and cons of antioxidant supplementation.

The Antioxidant-Cholesterol Link

As mentioned earlier, antioxidants fight heart disease, as well as a number of other illnesses, by foiling the activity of free radicals. But antioxidants also may help boost "good" HDL cholesterol and help artery-clogging LDL cholesterol resist oxidation, a chemical process that researchers believe increases the likelihood that LDL will collect in the arteries.

"LDL is the major cholesterol-carrying molecule in the bloodstream," says Thomas Bersot, MD, PhD, clinical professor of medicine at the University of California, San Francisco. Oxidized LDL is more likely to be trapped by macrophages, a type of cell in the walls of the arteries. When LDL starts to collect inside the macrophages, it sets up a chemical chain reaction that can accelerate oxidation and other artery-clogging processes.

"The accumulation of LDL in the macrophages initiates the entire cascade of events in atherosclerosis," says Dr. Bersot. "If you can prevent LDL from oxidizing, you may reduce the risk of developing hardening of the arteries."

Antioxidants to the Rescue

A number of studies have demonstrated an association between a higher intake of antioxidant supplements—particularly vitamins C and E—and a lower risk of heart disease.

Researchers in the Health Professionals Study, conducted at Harvard Medical School and the Harvard School of Public Health, followed 40,000 healthy male health care workers for 4 years, tracking how many developed heart disease during that time. They found that the men who consumed the most vitamin E had a lower risk of heart disease. Men who took 100 IU or more of vitamin E for at least 2 years cut their risk of heart disease by 37 percent compared with men who did not take any supplements.

A parallel Harvard study evaluated more than 87,000 healthy female nurses for 8 years. Women who consumed the most vitamin E were found to have a 34 percent reduced risk of developing heart disease compared with women who consumed the least vitamin E. Women who had taken vitamin E supplements for at least 2 years had a 41 percent lower chance of developing coronary disease than those who hadn't taken supplements. And women who consumed the most beta-carotene had a 22 percent reduced risk of heart ailments compared with women who consumed the least.

Researchers at the University of California, Los Angeles, found that men who consumed the most vitamin C had a 45 percent reduced risk of dying of heart disease; women had a 25 percent reduction in risk. The researchers used data from the first National Health and Nutrition Examination Survey, which included information about the vitamin intakes of more than 11,000 people.

Pumping Up HDL

The studies above did not specifically explore the relationship between blood cholesterol levels and antioxidants, but other research has examined the possibility that antioxidants may help raise HDL cholesterol levels and interfere with the oxidation of LDL.

"Several studies have shown that if you progress from consuming a relatively low amount of vitamin C—below 60 milligrams a day—up to about 250 to 500 milligrams a day, you'll experience a dose-related increase in HDL cholesterol," says Jeffrey Blumberg, PhD, director of the Antioxidant Research Laboratory at the Jean Mayer USDA Human Nutrition Research Center on Aging at Tufts University in Boston. "This may account for some of the benefits of vitamin C in heart disease."

A study published by the New York Academy of Sciences in New York City, which compared the heart disease risks of 696 men and women ages 60 and over, found that consuming more than 180 milligrams of vitamin C a day—more than three times the Daily Value (DV)—was associated with higher HDL cholesterol and lower blood pressure levels than consuming less than the DV of vitamin C a day. And at the Human Nutrition Research Center on Aging at Tufts, researchers found that higher blood levels of vitamin C (ascorbic acid) were associated with elevated HDL cholesterol and lower LDL cholesterol in more than 1,200 people.

Researchers at the University of California, San Diego, conducted two studies to determine the effects of vitamin E and beta-carotene—used individually, in combination, and together with vitamin C—on the oxidation of LDL. In the first phase of the study, eight people consumed 60 milligrams of beta-carotene per day for 3 months. Then, for another 3 months, they added 1,600 IU of vitamin E a day to the beta-carotene. Finally, for another 3 months, the participants added 2,000 milligrams of vitamin C to the vitamin E and beta-carotene.

In the second phase of the study, the participants consumed only vitamin E supplements (1,600 IU a day) for 5 months. Researchers concluded that long-term use of vitamin E in high doses hindered the oxidation of LDL by 30 to 50 percent. Beta-carotene did not seem to affect LDL's resistance to oxidation.

Good Food Sources of Antioxidants

What do clams, kale, and cantaloupe have in common? They're all brimming with antioxidants. Here's a short list of antioxidant-rich fare.

Vitamin C	Vitamin E	Beta-Carotene
Broccoli	Asparagus	Apricots
Brussels sprouts	Cereal (fortified)	Cantaloupe
Cantaloupe	Kale	Carrots
Cauliflower	Liver	Mangoes
Clams	Nuts	Papaya
Grapefruit	Pumpkin seeds	Peaches
Green and red	Sunflower seeds	Spinach
peppers	Sweet potatoes	Sweet potatoes
Mangoes	Vegetable oil	Tomatoes
Oranges	Wheat germ	Yellow squash
Papaya	Whole grain products	
Potatoes		
Watermelon		

Food Before Supplements

Some researchers, including Dr. Blumberg, believe that the DVs—set at levels designed to prevent nutritional deficiencies—are too low to help fight disease. "Going by only the nutritional deficiency criteria, the DVs are absolutely correct," he says. "But if you ask, 'How much vitamin C do I need to reduce my risk of heart disease, cancer, or cataracts?' you'd get a much different answer than the DVs."

What's more, some people may find it difficult to even reach the DVs through diet alone, particularly now that the newest recommendations for Americans are to eat five to nine servings of fruits and vegetables every day.

Heart-Healthy Indulgences

Guacamole: The Great Green Fat Fighter

Next time you dine at a Mexican restaurant, pass up the sour cream in favor of the guacamole. Avocado, the main ingredient in guacamole, is a very rich source of the antioxidant glutathione. Tests conducted at Louisiana State University showed that glutathione can help to block the absorption of harmful fat in the intestinal tract. It also protects the DNA in cells from free radical damage, which has been linked to aging. Avocados contain at least three times more glutathione than any other fruit.

Avocados are also high in unsaturated fat, and the U.S. government's dietary guidelines suggest that a diet based on moderate amounts of foods high in unsaturated fats can also help keep cholesterol low and offer some protection against heart disease.

Don't kid yourself, though: Eating too much fat of any kind means eating more calories than you need. Also, avocado can't completely combat the effects of the saturated fat from the refried beans and deep-fried chips in your Mexican meal.

To benefit your waistline and your heart, use the following strategies.

- When you make guacamole at home, cut the fat by using tomatillos (Mexican green tomatoes) in place of some of the avocados.

- Eat less of other fatty foods while you're enjoying your guacamole.

Though the results of antioxidant supplementation on heart health have been mixed, Dr. Blumberg says that they might help, and no harm can come from taking vitamin C and vitamin E at appropriate levels. He recommends consuming between 250 and 500 milligrams of vitamin C and between 100 and 200 IU of vitamin E in supplement form. These doses are safe, he says. Since taking large amounts of vitamin C has been reported to cause diarrhea, however, and high doses of vitamin E can cause an increased risk of death, be sure to check with your doctor before taking antioxidant supplements. Because supplements can't compensate for bad dietary habits, it's crucial to follow a healthy diet rich in fruits, vegetables, whole grains, low-fat or fat-free dairy products, and small amounts of meat, poultry, and fish. "Rather than relying on supplements, eat foods rich in antioxidants," says Dr. Bersot. "They'll provide antioxidant vitamins as well as other nutritional substances that may be beneficial."

See also Flavonoids

Apples

Benefits That Are More Than Skin Deep

An apple a day . . . has become more than cliché.

You've heard about this fruit that "keeps the doctor away" for so long that you probably take it for granted. But as it turns out, this claim is backed by cutting-edge scientific research. Numerous studies now indicate that apples can lower cholesterol and protect the heart in a couple of ways.

The Proof Is in the Pectin

Researchers have known for decades that apples are a good source of fiber. And that still holds true: A 5-ounce apple with the skin provides about 3 grams. But apples have one particular type of fiber, called pectin, that seems to specifically help lower cholesterol.

"Pectin is a soluble fiber that helps draw cholesterol out of the system," says Audrey Cross, PhD, associate clinical professor at Columbia University's Institute of Human Nutrition in New York City. The average apple contains 1.08 grams of pectin.

The benefits of pectin and apple's other sources of fiber have held up well to clinical research. In a study conducted by David L. Gee, PhD, professor of food science and nutrition at Central Washington University in Ellensburg, 26 men with elevated cholesterol (ranging from 200 to 255 milligrams/deciliter, or mg/dl) were divided into two groups. The first group ate three cookies with added apple fiber per day. These cookies contained a total of 14.5 grams of fiber, an amount equal to that found in four to five apples. The second group ate regular cookies. Otherwise, the men ate what they always ate.

After 6 weeks, in the group that ate the fiber-laden cookies, total cholesterol dropped an average of 15 points, or 7 percent. No improvements were seen in the placebo group.

In a follow-up study conducted by Dr. Gee and graduate student Karen Spencer, 25 men with cholesterol levels ranging from 200 to 270 mg/dl drank 20 ounces a day of FiberRich, a commercial apple juice brimming with pectin. After 6 weeks, the men's total cholesterol levels dipped an average of 10 percent, and their LDL cholesterol fell an average of 14 percent.

Other studies have pointed to apples' ability to lower blood cholesterol levels. In a French study, 30 healthy men and women added two to three apples to their diets each day for a month. Total cholesterol fell in 80 percent of the participants, by an average of 14 percent. One person's cholesterol plummeted 29 percent! HDL cholesterol, the "good" kind, rose slightly as well.

The Force of Flavonoids

The other way that apples protect the heart is with flavonoids, antioxidant compounds that protect the body from the damage of free radicals and "bad" LDL cholesterol. One type of flavonoid that's abundant in apples is quercetin, which is found in large amounts (about 4 milligrams per apple) in the apple's skin.

Quercetin seems to be a major player among antioxidants when it comes to heart health. In one study in Finland, people who got more quercetin in their diets over a 20-year period had a 20 percent lower risk of heart disease than those who got the least. A study in the Netherlands showed that men who ate an apple a day, along with 2 tablespoons of onions and four cups of tea, had a 32 percent lower risk of heart attack than those who ate fewer apples.

The Not-So-Forbidden Fruit

Perhaps the simplest way to take advantage of apples' power to pare blood cholesterol is to eat the raw fruit itself, say experts. "A fresh apple is a great snack food," says Evelyn Tribole, RD, a dietitian in Beverly Hills, California, and author of *Healthy Homestyle Cooking*. Try to choose fresh apples over juice. Though apple juice contains a bit of iron and a small amount of potassium, it gets stripped of most of its fiber and quercetin by the time it becomes juice. Plus, some brands have added sugar. So while apple juice is obviously a better choice than a soft drink, it still can't hold a candle to a fresh apple.

But there are other ways to enjoy the delicious taste of apples. Try these suggestions.

Heart-Healthy Indulgences

Apple Pie: A Delicious Way to Benefit from Pectin

A lot of evidence suggests that apples can help cut blood cholesterol, thanks to a sticky substance called pectin. Found in some fruits and vegetables, pectin is a soluble fiber that's thought to draw cholesterol out of the system. But apples are also full of flavonoids, which are the chemicals that appear to block the process that allows harmful LDL cholesterol to clog up your arteries.

So help yourself to a slice of apple pie every now and then. Just be sure to leave some of the crust on your plate—it may be loaded with shortening, a hydrogenated fat that's bad for your arteries.

If you want to cut the fat in your homemade piecrust, here are some tips.

Use less shortening. Although many pastry recipes tend to be fairly exact, it is often possible to cut the amount of shortening by about one-third without having a big impact on the texture of the crust.

Replace it with oil. If you use canola or safflower oil in place of some of the solid shortening, you'll be exchanging some of the saturated fat for a more heart-healthy monounsaturated or polyunsaturated fat.

• Mix sliced apples with a low-fat cheese, sprinkle with fresh chives, and serve on romaine lettuce. You might also toss sliced apples with raisins, almonds, and cooked chicken and splash the salad with tarragon vinegar.

• Add apples to baked goods. "You can grate apples into almost anything that you bake, including low-fat muffins and cakes," says Tribole. Try grating one large apple into a recipe that yields six large muffins.

• Sauté a side dish. Sautéed apples are a delicious accompaniment to meat (preferably leaner cuts). After sautéing turkey cutlets, for example, remove the meat from the pan and add sliced, peeled apples to the meat juices. Sauté the apples for 5 minutes, then stir in ½ cup of apple juice and cook until the apples are soft (about 3 minutes). Serve with the cutlets.

• Bake a guilt-free pastry. Chop up some apples, add cinnamon and a little sugar, wrap the apples in phyllo dough and bake, suggests Tribole. "You'll end up with something like apple strudel that's very low in fat," she says.

• Think "brown isn't bad." When it comes to choosing apples, your initial impulse might be to avoid varieties that brown easily. But in reality, the compounds that make apples brown are the same ones that provide heart-healthy benefits. So steer clear of apples that are bred to not brown, such as Granny Smith, in favor of other varieties.

To keep apples crisp, wrap them in a plastic bag and store them in the refrigerator. Apples kept at room temperature soften 10 times faster than refrigerated fruit.

Artichokes
Funny Food—Fantastic Results

In Renaissance times, the artichoke's reputation was somewhat scandalous—it was widely considered to be a powerful aphrodisiac.

Time and history have shown that artichokes really don't do much for your libido. But this strange vegetable, which is actually the immature flower of a thistle plant, may be an effective therapy for lowering cholesterol levels.

In a German study published in 2001, men and women who had high levels of total cholesterol (more than 280 milligrams/deciliter) received either 1,800 milligrams of dried artichoke extract or a placebo (an inactive pill) every day for 6 weeks. By the study's end, those who took the extract lowered their cholesterol by an average of 18 percent. The placebo group's cholesterol dropped by about 8 percent.

But that wasn't the only benefit. Researchers also found that levels of

Green Beans with Peppers and Artichokes

Makes 4 servings

- 12 ounces small red potatoes
- 8 ounces green beans
- 1 cup chopped roasted red bell peppers
- 8 water-packed artichoke hearts, halved
- $\frac{1}{3}$ cup tarragon vinegar
- 1 tablespoon olive oil
- 1 teaspoon Dijon mustard
- 1 clove garlic, minced
- $\frac{1}{2}$ teaspoon dried marjoram
- $\frac{1}{4}$ teaspoon ground black pepper
- $\frac{1}{4}$ teaspoon Worcestershire sauce

In a large saucepan, bring 1" of water to a boil. Place the potatoes on a steaming rack and set the rack in the pan. Cover and steam for 15 minutes, or until tender. Set aside to cool. When the potatoes are cool enough to handle, slice thinly and place in a large bowl.

In a medium saucepan, blanch the beans in boiling water for 5 minutes. Drain and add to the potatoes. Add the peppers and artichokes and toss to combine.

In a small bowl, whisk together the vinegar, oil, mustard, garlic, marjoram, black pepper, and Worcestershire sauce. Pour over the vegetables and toss to combine.

Per serving: 172 calories, 5.8 g fat (30% of calories), 3.7 g protein, 30.5 g carbohydrates, 0 mg cholesterol, 2.1 g dietary fiber, 113 mg sodium "bad" LDL cholesterol fell more than 20 percent in the people who took the extract and that their ratio of protective HDL to LDL also improved.

How does this extract help "choke" cholesterol? Artichokes contain a compound called cynarin, which increases production of bile by the liver. Studies also show that the extract boosts the flow of bile from the gallbladder. Bile plays a key role in the excretion of excess cholesterol from the body.

Artichoke leaf extract is available in pill form from a number of health food stores, as well as online sources. The supplement does not appear to have any adverse side effects, but it's best to stick to the recommended dosage, and, as with any supplement, speak with your doctor before using it.

Also, if you'd like to enjoy artichokes with your meals, you can team them up with other vegetables to create a side dish that can help you to reap the cholesterol-cutting benefits and taste of artichokes plus the heart-healthy benefits of olive oil. (See the recipe on the opposite page for one possibility.)

Avocados
Forbidden Fruit No More

If somebody told you that a fruit with 730 calories and up to 30 grams of fat was good for your heart, you'd probably say, "Yeah, right."

Yet amazingly, that's exactly the case with avocados. Despite their whopping calorie and fat numbers, these delicious fruits have been shown to lower total cholesterol, drop triglycerides, and maintain or even slightly raise levels of "good" HDL cholesterol.

How do they do it? Avocados are high in monounsaturated fat, which is known to reduce LDL, or "bad," cholesterol, and is especially rich in oleic acid, the same cholesterol-busting monounsaturated fat found in olive and canola oils.

Of course, the catch with avocados is that even a "good" fat like monounsaturated fat can be bad in high doses. But if you eat them occasionally, you might just chip a few points off your cholesterol count—and have some delicious dishes in the process.

Send Cholesterol South with This Southern Fruit

The connection between avocados and lower blood cholesterol began with a hunch: A team of Australian researchers suspected the link and decided to test their theory. In this study, 15 women alternated between a low-fat, high-carbohydrate diet (21 percent fat calories) and an avocado–enriched diet (36 percent fat calories) in which they ate from ½ to 1½ avocados per day.

After 3 weeks on the avocado-rich diet, the women's total cholesterol fell from an average of 236 to 217 milligrams/deciliter, or 8.2 percent, compared with 4.9 percent after 3 weeks on the low-fat plan. More significantly, however, "good" HDL cholesterol plummeted an average of 14 percent on the low-fat plan and not at all on the avocado diet. As a result, the ratio of total cholesterol to HDL increased 10.4 percent in the women on the low-fat plan but decreased 14.9 percent in the avocado eaters.

Other studies have shown further heart-healthy benefits of avocados. A study in Mexico of 16 women with diabetes showed that avocados lowered triglyceride levels by 20 percent. This is good news for people with diabetes, who typically have trouble keeping triglyceride levels down.

Another way avocados help your heart is with their high fiber content. Fiber helps shuttle cholesterol out of the body through your waste, and one avocado packs more fiber than a bran muffin: 10 grams, or about 40 percent of the Daily Value. Plus, avocados contain about 548 milligrams of potassium, 16 percent of the Daily Value and about 15 percent more than you get from a banana. Potassium has other heart-healthy properties, such as lowering blood pressure and reducing the risk of heart attack or stroke.

Get Monos in Moderation

Avocados contain zero dietary cholesterol, which is found only in animal-derived foods such as eggs, milk, and meats. But don't gobble avocados with abandon: About 71 to 88 percent of this fruit's calories come from fat. "Using one-eighth of an average avocado in a salad adds about 5 grams of fat," says Janet Lepke-Harris, RD, a dietitian in Charlotte, North Carolina, and a spokesperson for the American Dietetic Association.

A good way to incorporate avocado into your diet is to use it to replace foods high in saturated fat, like egg yolks, whole milk, and meats. That way, you're replacing bad fats with good, rather than adding more fat to an already fatty diet.

A Little Goes a Long Way

Many people stud their salads with chunks of avocado or add a few slices of the fruit to a sandwich. Here are a few additional tips for serving avocado, as well as advice on when and how to buy them.

• If possible, choose avocados from Florida instead of California. They have about two-thirds of the calories and half the fat.

• Another way to get avocados with less fat is to buy those harvested between November and March. They often have one-third the fat of those picked in September and October.

• The next time you make potato salad, use less mayonnaise and add some mashed avocado instead. You'll consume less saturated fat and dietary cholesterol and more heart-healthy monounsaturated fat.

• Slice an avocado in half, remove the seed, and stuff the fruit with chicken, seafood, or pasta salad prepared with low-fat or cholesterol-free mayo. To keep the avocado from turning brown, rub the flesh with a little lemon juice.

Note: If you buy avocados that aren't yet ripe enough to eat, you can speed up the ripening process by putting them in a paper bag and setting them aside for a few days.

See also Fiber

Beans

A Heart Saver from Down South

The growing Hispanic population in America today presents an interesting heart-health case study. Data seem to indicate that Mexicans have a lower incidence of heart disease, stroke, and high blood pressure than most American populations. Meanwhile, Hispanic Americans have rates of heart disease and high blood pressure that mirror those of white and black American populations—and they have an even higher incidence of high blood cholesterol.

Some researchers think they know part of the reason that this is occurring. Hispanics entering this country are ignoring a core component of their native diet—beans. And the evidence suggests that not only Hispanics, but all of us, would do well to get more of these tasty legumes.

Beans seem to help your heart in a number of ways. First, they are a great source of soluble fiber. "The soluble fiber found in beans and lentils lowers blood glucose responses, stabilizes blood sugar, and slows the absorption of fat from the intestine," says David L. Katz, MD, MPH, director of the Yale-Griffin Prevention Research Center in Derby, Connecticut, and author of *Dr. David Katz's Flavor-Full Diet*. "The net effect is to cause more cholesterol to leave the body through the intestines, lowering blood levels."

Second, they're high in protein and low in fat. This makes them a great alternative to other protein sources high in saturated fat, like red meat or whole-milk dairy products.

What's more, the fat that beans do have is the kind that you want in your diet. "Beans contain omega-3 fatty acids and loads of calcium," says Neal Barnard, MD, president of the Physicians Committee for Responsible Medicine in Washington, D.C. Omega-3 fatty acids, which are also found in certain fatty fish, have been shown in numerous studies to help prevent cardiovascular disease.

Beans' nutritional pedigree and culinary versatility mean they're perfect in virtually any dish, from fiery chili to savory soups. Best of all, whipping up quick, healthy bean dishes can be as simple as opening a can. Want more good reasons to pile your plate with beans? Read on.

The Benefits of Beans

A number of studies seem to support the notion that beans of all types are good for your heart. At the University of Kentucky in Lexington, one study showed that men with high cholesterol who added 1½ cups of pinto and navy beans a day to their diets saw their total cholesterol fall by 56 points on average after just 3 weeks. And in a separate study, 28 men who added an 8-ounce can of beans in tomato sauce to their diet every day saw cholesterol drop by 10.4 percent and triglycerides plunge by 10.8 percent after 3 weeks.

Researchers in New Zealand put 40 people with high cholesterol on a low-fat diet to which either cooked beans or oat bran was added. These folks' total cholesterol declined slightly on both diets. But their "good" HDL cholesterol rose significantly when they ate the beans rather than the oat bran.

And in Costa Rica, a Harvard University study of more than 2,000 individuals showed that those who ate one serving of black beans once a day were 38 percent less likely to suffer from a heart attack than those who ate beans less than once a month.

The Basics of Bean Cookery

Beans warrant a prominent place on your menu. These tips can get you started.

• If you want to use dried whole beans, you'll need to soak them. Put them in cold water overnight, so they'll be ready to cook the next day. Or try the quick soak method: Boil the beans for 2 minutes, then set them aside to soak for an hour or so.

• To bypass soaking, opt for lentils, suggests Dr. Katz. "Lentils are rich in many nutrients, especially soluble fiber and high-quality protein," he says. "They have a low glycemic load and make an excellent substitute for meat. Try them in lentil soup, in stews, or in lentil salads in the summer."

• Add canned beans to soups, salads, and casseroles. Rinse the beans to remove excess sodium.

• To give stews a fiber boost, add a can of chickpeas, kidney beans, lima beans, or black beans.

• Enjoy burritos made with beans instead of beef, suggests Dr. Barnard. "There's nothing better than a homemade bean burrito with jalapeños," he says. Top it with salsa, diced tomatoes, or shredded lettuce.

Can't Beat These Beans

Want to add fiber power to your cholesterol-lowering diet? Load up on these legumes.

Legume (½ cup cooked)	Soluble Fiber (g)
Kidney beans	2.8
Cranberry beans	2.7
Lima beans	2.7
Black beans	2.4
Navy beans	2.2
Lentils	2.0
Pinto beans	1.9
Great Northern beans	1.4
Chickpeas	1.3
Split peas	1.1

• Mix any type of mashed canned beans with chopped onions, fresh garlic, and low-sodium tamari (a kind of soy sauce). Spread the mixture on crackers or spoon into taco shells.

• Add a trickle of olive oil and some fresh garlic to mashed canned chickpeas and spread on your favorite bread.

• Explore the ways different cultures use beans. You might try making a spicy Cuban black bean soup; Middle Eastern hummus (a savory spread of chickpeas, lemon juice, garlic, and fresh mint, served with pita bread); Italian *pasta e fagioli* (pasta with beans); or Southern-style hoppin' John (black-eyed peas and rice—hold the ham).

• If you're dining in a Mexican restaurant, avoid refried beans, says Martin Yadrick, RD, a dietitian in Manhattan Beach, California, and a spokesperson for the American Dietetic Association. "Traditional refried beans are prepared with lard," he says. "Ask for pinto beans or black beans, which contain a minimal amount of fat."

Degassing Legumes

Beans can cause gastrointestinal distress in some people. The gas-producing culprits: stachyose and raffinose, sugars that are the by-products of beans, says

Linda Van Horn, PhD, RD, professor of preventive medicine at Northwestern University Feinberg School of Medicine in Chicago. To help prevent gas, "soak beans overnight or for several hours before you cook them, and discard the water they've been soaking in," advises Dr. Van Horn. "Soaking beans breaks down some of these sugars."

You might also consider trying Beano. This over-the-counter product really does help reduce gas in some people, according to a study conducted at the University of California, San Diego. Folks who consumed eight drops of Beano after the first bite of a meal of meatless chili seemed to experience fewer gas eruptions than those who had taken a placebo (an inactive liquid), according to the participants' self-reported symptoms.

See also Fiber, Fish, Fish Oil Supplements

Berries

Little "Jewels" of Heart Health

In years past, turning to the government for dietary advice generally yielded pretty tame recommendations, such as "eat more fruits and vegetables."

Lately, however, you may have noticed that they're getting a little more descriptive with this advice. Turn to the American Heart Association's Web site, for example, and now the recommendation is to eat more of the "deeply colored" fruits and vegetables.

Why the specificity? As it turns out, darker and brighter fruits and vegetables tend to have more vitamins, minerals, and antioxidant compounds, which means they're better for your heart. And popular berries like blackberries, blueberries, raspberries, cranberries, and strawberries fall squarely into this category of antioxidant-rich fruits.

The Benefits of Berries

We've known for years that berries are a delicious seasonal treat. But it's only recently that a growing amount of evidence has shown just how good they are for you, too. In 2006, a group of researchers tried to measure the antioxidant content of more than 1,000 common foods. When this table was broken down by serving size, five of the top 10 foods that are richest in antioxidants were berries. This included blackberries at number one, strawberries at number three, cranberries at number five, raspberries at number seven, and blueberries at number nine.

Along with their incredible antioxidant potential, berries are brimming with other healthy vitamins and minerals, including folate, fiber, and potassium. "In an analysis of data from large dietary studies in the United States, strawberry eaters had higher intake and serum levels of folate, higher intake of fiber and vitamin C, lower homocysteine levels, and lower blood pressure than non–strawberry eaters," says Jaime Schwartz, RD, a dietitian with the California Strawberry Commission. "Homocysteine is an amino acid in the blood that is considered to be an independent marker for heart disease risk."

What's more, adds Schwartz, berries might have a more direct effect on cholesterol by preventing the oxidation of LDL cholesterol. In research at the University of California, Los Angeles, "strawberry extracts of both low and high concentrations inhibited the oxidation of human LDL cholesterol cells in culture by 54 percent and 86 percent, respectively," she says. "Oxidation of LDL is a key step in the process of atherosclerosis, the accumulation of plaque on artery walls that can lead to cardiovascular disease."

Strawberries aren't the only cholesterol-fighting berries either. Another study seems to indicate that an antioxidant compound found in blueberries, pterostilbene, may lower cholesterol as effectively as the commercial cholesterol drug ciprofibrate, which is sold under the name Lipanor. Though it's unclear exactly how many blueberries you'd need to eat to gain maximum benefit, this study is just one more reason why it's a good idea to chow down on tasty berries.

Be Supermarket Strawberry Savvy

Have a tough time getting great-tasting berries at the grocery store? "I prefer strawberries with a little bit of a white shoulder," says Erik Jertberg, a strawberry grower in California. "I've found that just before they reach 100 percent maturity, the berries are a little sweeter, a little juicier, and may even last longer. The ones that don't look quite ripe enough are often the sweetest."

Then, once you get those berries home, Jertberg says it's easy to get them ready to eat. "Keep them in the fridge until you are ready to eat them, then wash them, and bring them up to room temperature," he says. "These three easy steps will give you the best eating experience."

"Berry" Delicious

This is but a small sampling of the hard science behind berries. Of course, if you're trying to eat for your heart, berries have another thing going for them that many other "health" foods don't—they're absolutely delicious, so you don't exactly have to twist any arms to get people to eat them. Still, the California Strawberry Commission has come up with a list of creative ways to enjoy not only strawberries but also other berries in your diet.

• Think outside the cereal bowl. Breakfast is a great meal for enjoying berries, and you can do a lot more than just add them to cereal. "Spread low-fat cream cheese on a whole grain English muffin, and top it with sliced strawberries for a sweet and creamy breakfast you can take on the go," says Schwartz. "Or make a smoothie with low-fat soy milk, frozen or fresh berries, honey, and ginger. You could also make a parfait with sliced berries, vanilla yogurt, and low-fat granola."

• Add them to salad. Looking for an unorthodox way to enjoy berries? Mix them up with greens and other ingredients in a refreshing summer salad. Schwartz recommends starting with a base of leafy greens such as spinach, romaine, or red lettuce, and then adding strawberries and items such as sunflower seeds, almonds, turkey, chicken, or steak for texture and flavor. "You can also make a strawberry vinaigrette to give your salad some added zing," she says.

• Dress up an entrée. You can make an average main dish a lot more interesting by topping chicken or salmon with a strawberry mango salsa, adding strawberries to chicken and shrimp kebabs, or using fresh berries as a fish topper, says Schwartz.

• Keep desserts healthy. Instead of ice cream, try fresh berries over vanilla yogurt with chopped nuts and granola, says Schwartz. Or prepare a cheese plate with a variety of fresh berries. And finally, dip strawberries in dark chocolate for a delicious one-two punch of antioxidant potential. Dark chocolate, like the strawberry itself, is rich in antioxidants. Just make sure not to overdo the chocolate.

Broccoli

A Star among Veggies

When it comes to your heart, vegetables are always a good food choice. But for whatever reason, some vegetables have certain intangible qualities that make them rise above the pack. Based on the most recent research, it's safe to say that broccoli is one of these vegetables. "Broccoli is one of the healthiest foods that you can possibly eat," says Christopher Gardner, PhD, of the Stanford Prevention Research Center at Stanford University Medical Center.

Just what makes broccoli so special? For starters, it's like a multivitamin in natural food form. Name a nutrient—vitamin C, vitamin A, soluble fiber, calcium, potassium, folate—chances are broccoli will give you a healthy dose of it.

And medical trials seem to indicate that it heals, too. For years, broccoli has shown itself to be a proven cancer fighter. Now, research is finding that broccoli might fight heart disease in a similar fashion. Researchers at the University of Saskatchewan fed broccoli sprouts to rats with a risk of high blood pressure and stroke. After 14 weeks, the rats that were eating the sprouts had lower blood pressure and decreased inflammation of the heart and kidneys.

Scientists believe that the antioxidant compound glucoraphanin is the ingredient in broccoli sprouts that reduces inflammation and might prevent heart disease. Though human trials are still needed, the researchers estimate that adults could receive a similar benefit by eating just 2 to 4 ounces of broccoli sprouts with a meal. (Broccoli sprouts have a good deal more glucoraphanin than broccoli itself.)

Better Bites of Broccoli

Unfortunately, broccoli is one of those veggies that make some people turn up their noses. But there are ways to make it more interesting in meals. Here's how:

• Make broccoli a breakfast ingredient in an egg-white omelet, along with other healthy ingredients like onions, spinach, and tomatoes.

• Simply serve broccoli florets raw along with carrots, celery sticks, and a bit of low-fat veggie dip.

• Mix broccoli with pasta sauce and serve it over whole wheat noodles.

• Use broccoli florets as a healthy pizza topping, along with tomato sauce and a bit of low-fat cheese.

• Add cut-up broccoli florets or broccoli sprouts to salads, and sprinkle broccoli sprouts on sandwiches with whole grain bread and lean meat or tuna.

Calcium

Not Just for Bone Health

Thanks in large part to the hard work of the National Dairy Council, calcium is known prominently for its role in building strong, healthy bones.

Though this is the mineral's most famous (and most well-researched) role, it's by no means the only part that calcium plays in the health of our bodies. In fact, calcium seems to have a significant impact on our heart health as well.

The most clear evidence that calcium helps our hearts seems to be in the area of high blood pressure. Studies have shown that a calcium deficiency can lead to high blood pressure and calcium supplementation has reduced blood pressure in those who have high blood pressure.

Though more research is needed, a few recent studies seem to indicate that calcium plays a role in lowering cholesterol as well. Read on to see how.

How Calcium Might Quash Cholesterol

Though researchers have suspected the link between calcium and cholesterol since the 1950s, initial studies weren't that promising. But recently, studies have looked more specifically at how calcium affects the separate components of cholesterol, such as LDL (the "bad" kind) and HDL (the "good" kind).

This specificity has yielded more promising results. And the news appears to be good for both men and women and for increasing calcium intake through both food and supplements.

Researchers at the University of Texas Southwestern Medical Center at Dallas put 13 men with moderately high cholesterol on either a high-calcium diet (2,200 milligrams of calcium per day) or a low-calcium diet (410 milligrams of calcium per day) for 10 weeks. For the next 10 weeks, the men resumed their regular diets. During the study's final 10 weeks, the men who first consumed the high-calcium diet followed the low-calcium plan, and vice versa.

The researchers found that the men's total cholesterol fell an average of 6 percent on the high-calcium diet. Even more significantly, their LDL cholesterol dropped an average of 11 percent. Since experts generally agree that every 1 percent decrease in LDL cholesterol results in a 2 percent decrease in heart disease risk, the participants' risk dropped over 20 percent.

Along with the encouraging study results of adding more calcium to the diet, a study performed at the University of Auckland in New Zealand showed that calcium supplementation may benefit cholesterol levels. This time, 223 postmenopausal women took part in a study in which they either took a calcium citrate supplement or a placebo (an inactive pill). The women in the test group took two 200-milligram tablets in the morning before breakfast and three 200-milligram tablets in the evening.

After 12 months of this routine, the women taking the calcium supplements experienced an average 7 percent increase in their levels of "good" HDL cholesterol. The researchers were encouraged by the findings, and similar tests on men are scheduled for the near future.

How might calcium reduce cholesterol? According to the University of Texas study, calcium may both block the absorption of saturated fat and bind with cholesterol-containing bile acids in the digestive system. The body then excretes these acids, giving excess cholesterol the boot, too. In fact, the men in the University of Texas study excreted 13 percent saturated fat while following the high-calcium diet, compared with only 6 percent while on the low-calcium plan.

Fat-Free Ways to Bone Up Your Diet

Whether the link between increased calcium consumption and lower blood cholesterol will be borne out by further study remains to be seen. Still, "there are many good reasons to increase your calcium intake," says Robert P. Heaney, MD, professor of medicine at Creighton University School of Medicine in Omaha, Nebraska, and an expert on calcium.

The most crucial reason? Many people simply don't get enough of this vital mineral. In fact, the Surgeon General's 2004 report on "Bone Health and Osteoporosis" stressed exactly that point. The optimum intake is 1,000 milligrams a day for women ages 25 to 50, menopausal women (ages 51 to 65) who take estrogen, and men ages 25 to 65. That amount jumps to 1,500 milligrams a day for menopausal women who don't take estrogen and for all men and women over age 65. Yet it's estimated that 50 percent of women over age 35 consume less than 600 milligrams of calcium a day—far less than they need.

Fortunately, it's easy to fortify your heart and bones with calcium. Simply consume more low-fat or fat-free milk, yogurt, and cheese, which contain all of the calcium of whole-milk dairy products with fewer calories. Other good sources of calcium include sardines and canned salmon, calcium-fortified orange juice, and leafy green vegetables, particularly bok choy and collards.

Calculate Your Calcium Quota

Chances are you won't find a single-dose multivitamin/mineral supplement that contains 100 percent of the optimal amount of 1,000 milligrams of calcium. And if you're a woman over age 50 or a man over age 65, you need even more calcium: 1,500 milligrams per day (150 percent of the Daily Value). So you may want to consider taking a calcium supplement. Here's how to find out if you're giving your heart and bones enough of this essential nutrient.

1. Determine your calcium goal.

2. Next, subtract 300 milligrams for each serving of milk, yogurt, cheese, or calcium-fortified orange juice that you typically consume each day.

3. Subtract any calcium that you may get from a multivitamin/mineral supplement. Most supplements contain 200 milligrams or less.

If, after your calculations, you're coming up short of your calcium goal, you need to take a calcium supplement, says William P. Castelli, MD, a cardiologist at the Heart Center of MetroWest in Framingham, Massachusetts, and former director of the Framingham Heart Study.

Choosing a Supplement

If you suspect that you're not getting enough calcium through your diet, you might consider taking calcium supplements, available in drugstores and health food stores, says Dr. Heaney. The most common supplements contain calcium carbonate, but calcium citrate is also a good choice that might be easier for some people to absorb than calcium carbonate.

The following guidelines can help you choose calcium supplements properly, says Dr. Heaney.

• Take calcium supplements in small doses—500 milligrams or less at a time.

• Take calcium supplements with meals to ensure good absorption, says Dr. Heaney. He recommends chewable supplements: "They disintegrate best," he says. Avoid "natural source" calcium carbonate supplements made from bonemeal, dolomite, or oyster shell, however. Some studies indicate that these products may contain unhealthy amounts of lead and other heavy metals.

• Make sure to get the Daily Value of vitamin D (400 IU): It's essential for calcium absorption. Consume foods fortified with vitamin D, including fat-free milk and some breads and cereals. Or consider taking a daily multivitamin/mineral supplement that meets 100 percent of your daily vitamin D requirement.

• Try to avoid calcium supplements that contain aluminum. This chemical can deplete the body's supply of phosphate, which it needs to absorb calcium, says Dr. Heaney. "But if you have a peptic ulcer and need to take supplements that contain aluminum, make sure you get extra calcium," he advises.

• Don't take calcium supplements with high-fiber wheat bran cereals: These cereals can reduce calcium absorption by 25 percent or more.

• Drink lots of water to help avoid constipation, a possible side effect of calcium supplements.

Supplements are not a substitute for a low-fat diet or cholesterol-lowering drugs (if your doctor has prescribed them), says Dr. Heaney. But "if you're eating a low-fat, low–saturated fat, low-cholesterol diet, some additional calcium may be helpful," he says. "Women might want an extra 1,000 milligrams a day of calcium—it can also help protect against osteoporosis." For men, taking an additional 800 milligrams of calcium over the optimal amounts may be sufficient.

While research indicates that calcium does not heighten the risk of kidney stone formation, if you have kidney stones, it's still a good idea to check with your doctor before taking calcium supplements. In fact, says Dr. Heaney, "a high-calcium diet actually protects against the absorption of oxalic acid, the principal risk factor in the formation of most kidney stones."

Canola Oil

The Lightest Oil of All

Ask a sampling of people what the healthiest cooking oil is, and the answer will invariably be olive oil.

Their praise is not unwarranted—olive oil is a rich source of monounsaturated fat, which has been shown in multiple studies to lower levels of "bad" LDL cholesterol, while at the same time leaving levels of "good" HDL cholesterol alone or slightly raising them. It's certainly a better choice than coconut oil, which is positively brimming with cholesterol-boosting saturated fat. And while safflower and corn oils contain polyunsaturated fat rather than saturated fat, this type of fat typically lowers not only bad cholesterol but also good cholesterol.

While olive oil seems to be getting all the good ink these days, it's not the only oil that should be on your heart-health shopping list. The other one—which may not be as famous but may be just as good for your heart—is canola oil.

Promising Results

A number of studies have shown that canola oil can be effective in reducing elevated cholesterol. For example, at the Kenneth L. Jordan Heart Foundation and Research Center in Montclair, New Jersey, and Elmhurst General

Hospital in Queens, New York, 36 people with either high blood cholesterol or high blood pressure added 1 ounce (about 2 tablespoons) of canola oil to their diets per day, using it in place of other oils and spreads. After 4 months, the participants' average total cholesterol fell from 254 to 248 milligrams/deciliter (mg/dl), and their LDL cholesterol dipped from 173 to 160 mg/dl. What's more, these folks' HDL cholesterol rose slightly, from 47 to 51 mg/dl.

Researchers at the University of Helsinki in Finland compared the effect on blood cholesterol of a diet high in monounsaturated fat and a diet high in polyunsaturated fat. For 2 weeks, the researchers fed 59 people a baseline diet that was high in saturated fat. Then the participants alternated between two diets—the first enriched with canola oil, and the second, with sunflower oil. Both diets supplied 38 percent of their calories as fat. But the sunflower oil diet was higher in polyunsaturated fat and lower in monounsaturated fat.

After 25 days on each diet, total cholesterol among men and women on the canola-enriched diet dropped 15 percent, and LDL cholesterol levels dipped 23 percent below the baseline level. By comparison, the total cholesterol of the sunflower oil group decreased 12 percent, and the LDL cholesterol fell 17 percent from the baseline. Neither diet affected levels of HDL cholesterol.

What about Olive Oil?

How does canola oil fare against olive oil? Though some experts prefer olive oil because it is a more natural oil (canola oil is extracted from heavily processed rapeseed oil), most agree that their health benefits are similar. Olive oil consists of almost 70 percent monounsaturated fats, but canola oil is close behind at 60 percent.

Though canola oil is lower in monounsaturated fat than olive oil, it is also lower in saturated fat. "Of the five vegetable oils lowest in saturated fat—canola, olive, corn, safflower, and sunflower—none is lower than canola," says Evelyn Tribole, RD, a dietitian in Beverly Hills, California, and author of *Healthy Homestyle Cooking*. "Canola oil contains 6 percent saturated fat, and olive oil, 15 percent saturated fat."

The bottom line? You can use both canola oil and olive oil as part of a heart-healthy diet. The best course of action, advises Tribole, is to replace the saturated fat in your diet, such as butter, with unsaturated fat, such as canola oil.

The Flavorless Advantage

Canola oil may have one other advantage over olive oil for some—it's nearly flavorless. That means for dishes where you want to taste the food and not the oil—such as stir-fries, sautéed vegetables, baked goods, sauces, and countless others—canola oil may be the oil of choice. And it's a healthier choice than other mostly flavorless oils such as safflower, corn, and vegetable oils.

Of course, olive oil still has its place in salad dressings and other recipes where you want its distinctive flavor. But when you don't, canola oil is a great alternative.

However you decide to use canola oil, keep it fresh. Oils high in monounsaturated fat tend to go bad faster than other oils. So if you haven't used up a bottle of canola oil about a month after opening it, store it in the refrigerator.

See also Olive Oil

Chocolate

Go for the Dark Stuff

Chocolate as a health food? This news just might be big enough to send waves of joy through the population at large. But that's exactly what the latest research has shown: Chocolate can increase levels of "good" HDL cholesterol, while leaving levels of the "bad" (LDL) at bay.

The reason for the sea change on chocolate is that it's positively overflowing with flavonoids, antioxidants that seem to neutralize the artery-clogging plaque that leads to a heart attack.

Researchers at Pennsylvania State University in University Park found that eating moderate amounts of chocolate as part of an overall healthy diet may indeed help your heart. "An ounce of dark chocolate contains 10 times more antioxidants than a strawberry," says Penny Kris-Etherton, PhD, RD, distinguished professor of nutrition at Penn State. "In addition, my preliminary research shows that a diet containing about an ounce of chocolate a day increases good cholesterol and prevents bad cholesterol from oxidizing, a process that may lead to heart disease."

Here's how you can sensibly enjoy the sweet benefits of chocolate.

• Think of chocolate as a fun, occasional part of a balanced diet. Its new image as a heart helper doesn't mean that you can have it with breakfast, lunch, and dinner. It does contain fat, and too much of that leads to higher cholesterol and weight gain.

• Opt for the dark stuff. "Dark chocolate has a high concentration of flavonoids, milk chocolate has much less, and white chocolate doesn't have any at all," says David L. Katz, MD, MPH, director of the Yale-Griffin Prevention Research Center in Derby, Connecticut, and author of *Dr. David Katz's Flavor-Full Diet*. "Assuming you make room for it in a diet that is not causing weight gain, one 3-ounce piece of dark chocolate with 60 percent cocoa is clearly heart healthy. More work is still needed to define the lower effective dose."

Chromium

Cholesterol Help That Really Shines

The word *chrome* brings to mind shiny hubcaps and bumpers—but the mineral that these things are made from, chromium, might shine even brighter when it comes to our heart health.

The majority of studies looking at the impact of chromium on our health have been in the area of diabetes. And here, the results look particularly promising. "Chromium is vital in diabetes, as it has been shown to help control blood sugar," says Fred Pescatore, MD, a traditionally trained physician practicing nutritional medicine and author of numerous books including, most recently, *The Hamptons Diet*. "It even has a qualified health claim by the Food and Drug Administration since 1996."

But diabetes isn't the only condition beneficially affected by chromium. Some studies indicate that chromium may boost the body's stores of "good"

HDL cholesterol. "When people who follow a normal diet—which tends to be marginally chromium-deficient—consume more chromium, their cholesterol and triglyceride levels benefit," says Richard A. Anderson, PhD, lead scientist at the USDA Human Nutrition Research Center in Beltsville, Maryland, and a leading expert on chromium.

The Cholesterol Connection

Researchers at Oklahoma State University in Stillwater had 21 people ages 60 and over take 150 micrograms of chromium every day for 3 months. Another 21 people took a placebo (an inactive pill).

Chromium takers with normal cholesterol exhibited no change in their cholesterol levels. But chromium takers with high cholesterol saw their total cholesterol go down 12 percent and their "bad" LDL cholesterol plummet 14 percent. Just as important, their levels of HDL cholesterol didn't change.

In a second study conducted at Oklahoma State University, researchers had 24 people ages 55 and over take one of three supplements: chromium (210 micrograms), copper, or zinc. After 2 months, the total cholesterol of the folks taking the chromium fell 12 points, from 217 to 205 milligrams/deciliter. When they stopped taking the chromium, their total cholesterol crept up again.

Copper and zinc had no effect on cholesterol levels.

In Jerusalem, 76 heart disease patients—about one-third of whom also had type 2 diabetes—consumed either a 250-microgram chromium supplement or a placebo every day for 7 to 16 months. The total cholesterol of the men in the chromium group didn't change. But their HDL cholesterol increased by 21 to 25 percent.

Though these studies are a few years old, Dr. Anderson adds that an animal study published in 2006 confirmed the link between low chromium levels and high cholesterol.

Getting Enough Chromium

The Daily Value for chromium is 120 micrograms. The average American man consumes 33 micrograms of the mineral a day, and the average woman, 25 micrograms.

Dr. Pescatore says that there is a good reason for this deficiency: "It's impossible to get enough from foods, as our soil has been depleted of chromium. The only other place to find it in high amounts in a food source is brewer's yeast, which most people will not eat."

That's why it's a good idea to take a multivitamin/mineral supplement to get an adequate intake of chromium every day. Dr. Anderson recommends taking one containing 50 to 200 micrograms of chromium. "One leading brand contains 100 micrograms of chromium," he says. "That extra 100 micrograms a day can serve as an insurance policy should there be a deficiency in your diet."

If you have diabetes, you may need even more chromium, says Dr. Anderson—about 400 to 600 micrograms a day. Is consuming this amount of chromium safe? Yes, says Dr. Anderson.

"We've been studying chromium for decades, and we've never documented a single case of a negative effect," he says. Still, check with your doctor before taking more than a 200-microgram supplement per day.

A Strike against Diabetes

As mentioned earlier, diabetes is the other condition that chromium can help control. And since people with diabetes run an increased risk of developing heart disease, this is another big benefit of the mighty mineral.

Most people with diabetes have glucose intolerance, a condition in which blood sugar levels are out of control. That's because insulin, a hormone that helps control blood sugar levels, doesn't work properly. Chromium particularly benefits people who already have diabetes by making insulin work more effectively.

In one study, Richard A. Anderson, PhD, lead scientist at the USDA Human Nutrition Research Center in Beltsville, Maryland, had 17 people—8 of whom had mild glucose intolerance—eat a chromium-poor diet. After a month, Dr. Anderson divided these people into two groups. While both groups continued on the low-chromium diet, the first group took 200 micrograms of chromium per day. The second group received a placebo (an inactive pill). Five weeks later, the groups were switched, with the first group receiving the placebo and vice versa.

The chromium supplements didn't affect blood sugar levels in the glucose-tolerant folks. But the blood sugar levels of the glucose-intolerant people rose nearly 50 percent less when they were taking chromium supplements than when they didn't take these supplements. The upshot? Chromium may reverse glucose intolerance, says Dr. Anderson.

Additionally, "there is some evidence that chromium also acts as an appetite suppressant," says David L. Katz, MD, MPH, director of the Yale-Griffin Prevention Research Center in Derby, Connecticut, and author of *Dr. David Katz's Flavor-Full Diet*. "Since weight loss is so important in controlling diabetes, this is a secondary way that the supplement can help."

As far as foods go, there's always brewer's yeast, if you can stomach it. Another option that can help is a popular breakfast cereal. "Total breakfast cereal is very high in chromium," says Dr. Anderson. "One serving contains nearly 27 micrograms of chromium, which is probably as much as you'll get from everything else you eat all day."

But you need to watch the rest of your diet, too, says Dr. Anderson—especially if you have a sweet tooth. Consuming too many highly processed, sugary foods can rob the body of chromium (which is excreted through the urine). According to Dr. Anderson, "eating lots of simple sugars may also increase your need for chromium supplements because you're consuming fewer chromium-rich foods. So you need to pay attention to your overall diet as well as to the amount of chromium you're getting."

Cinnamon

A Surprisingly Heart-Healthy Choice

Cinnamon is hardly what you think of as a health food. Of course, when you consider that the "cinnamon" in our diets is usually accompanied by the words "roll," "toast," or "bears" . . . well, it's easy to understand the skepticism.

Strip away all the fat, sugar, and calories of the items that cinnamon is flavoring, though, and what you're left with is one of the most potent antioxidant sources on the planet. In a 2006 survey of the antioxidant content of common foods in our diet, cinnamon came in at number four on the list when comparing the amount of antioxidants in 100 grams of each type of food.

And while cinnamon might not directly lower cholesterol levels (it is still being decided), Ann G. Kulze, MD, founder and CEO of Just Wellness, a wellness consulting firm in Mt. Pleasant, South Carolina, and the author of *Dr. Ann's 10-Step Diet,* says that it may help the body metabolize cholesterol and usher it out of the system more quickly. David L. Katz, MD, MPH, director of the Yale-Griffin Prevention Research Center in Derby, Connecticut, and author of *Dr. David Katz's Flavor-Full Diet,* adds that cinnamon can improve people's sensitivity to insulin, and it stabilizes blood sugar in the body. This makes it useful for people with diabetes as well.

The Studies on Cinnamon

Though more research is needed, the few small studies performed on cinnamon and heart health have had mixed results. The consensus so far seems to be that cinnamon does have a positive effect on blood sugar. But whether or not cinnamon can really reduce cholesterol and triglyceride levels is still up in the air.

The most promising results came from a 2003 study conducted in Pakistan. In this study, 60 people with type 2 diabetes were divided into six groups. They received either varying doses of cinnamon in capsule form (1 gram, 3 grams, or 6 grams) or a placebo (an inactive pill) for 40 days.

After the trial period was over, those taking the cinnamon experienced vast improvements across the board in their blood sugar (18 to 29 percent), triglycerides (23 to 30 percent), LDL cholesterol (7 to 27 percent), and total cholesterol (12 to 26 percent). The results at the time seemed to confirm that adding cinnamon to the diet can help with high cholesterol, at least in those with type 2 diabetes. Moreover, the participants in the study continued to see benefits up to 20 days after the cinnamon treatment had ceased.

According to researchers at the USDA, what makes cinnamon work is a flavonoid compound known as methylhydroxy chalcone polymer, or MHCP. Researchers theorize that this antioxidant activates the insulin receptors inside your cells, causing them to begin using up blood sugar for energy.

A more recent study completed in 2006 of 79 patients with type 2 diabetes who took either cinnamon extract or a placebo for 4 months noted a similar response to blood sugar levels. However, researchers did not see the same changes to cholesterol levels that were noted in the 2003 study.

Be Sensible with This Spice

If you're interested in adding cinnamon to your own heart-healthy regimen, it's best not to overdo it, as too much cinnamon might be toxic. That's why experts recommend sticking to a teaspoon or less daily. "This can be as simple as sprinkling it into your coffee, or onto a healthy dessert," says Dr. Katz. "There are also cinnamon supplements available, but the proper therapeutic dose is still a work in progress."

In the meantime, talk to your doctor if you have diabetes and are considering adding cinnamon to your diet. It may alter the effects of your existing insulin medication.

Also, you'll want to continue to steer clear of cinnamon rolls, muffins, and other fatty treats with cinnamon flavor. Remember: Just because it says "cinnamon" on the label doesn't mean it's healthy!

Coenzyme Q$_{10}$

The Heart Supplement

It's fitting that another name for coenzyme Q$_{10}$ is "ubiquinone," which comes from the term *ubiquitous*, meaning "everywhere." That's because the enzyme is found in every cell in the body. It's critical in producing energy for our cells, which makes it vital for a properly functioning body. "Coenzyme Q$_{10}$ is found in the highest concentrations in organs that have the highest metabolic energy requirements, such as the heart, kidneys, liver, and skeletal muscles," says Robert Barry, PhD, a former advisor to the National Institutes of Health and a member of the scientific affairs department of Kaneka Nutrients, a supplement manufacturer in Pasadena, Texas.

Coenzyme Q$_{10}$ has a second proven benefit to the body, says Dr. Barry. "Coenzyme Q$_{10}$ is one of the most powerful lipid–soluble antioxidants known, preventing the generation of free radicals as well as oxidative modifications to proteins, lipids, and DNA," he says. "Coenzyme Q$_{10}$ can also regenerate the active antioxidant forms of vitamin E and vitamin C."

So while coenzyme Q$_{10}$ doesn't specifically lower cholesterol, its antioxidant potential makes it critical for preventing free radicals from causing damage in the heart and arteries that can lead to heart disease, stroke, high blood pressure, and congestive heart failure.

Moreover, it's important to realize that levels of coenzyme Q$_{10}$ in the body decrease with age. That means the older you get, the more you might want to consider coenzyme Q$_{10}$ to help preserve your body's heart health, recommend our experts. "Supplementation of coenzyme Q$_{10}$ can replenish the diminished levels of Q$_{10}$, fostering a protective defense against oxidative stress and age-related disease," says Dr. Barry. Oxidative stress creates wear and tear on the heart and arteries.

A Heart Helper

Coenzyme Q$_{10}$ has been a drug for congestive heart failure in Japan since 1974, but it was not recommended for sale in the United States until 2001. Once approved, though, it quickly became a top 10 supplement in sales and has remained there ever since.

When you see the research on coenzyme Q$_{10}$ and the heart, it's easy to understand its popularity. Though much of the research has demonstrated its positive impact on congestive heart failure, coenzyme Q$_{10}$ has also been shown to improve the function of the arteries as well as protect them from the oxidative damage caused by cholesterol.

Coenzyme Q$_{10}$ has another indirect relationship to blood cholesterol as well. As more and more people are being prescribed statin drugs to control their cholesterol, studies seem to indicate that statins may cause a coenzyme Q$_{10}$ deficiency in the body. Thus, coenzyme Q$_{10}$ supplementation might be beneficial for those taking statin drugs to maintain healthy levels as well as preserve heart health.

How to Take It

Though doses of coenzyme Q$_{10}$ have varied quite a bit in studies of the supplement, the general range is anywhere from 30 to 300 milligrams daily, usually divided into two or three doses. It also helps to take the supplements with food to improve their absorption. And, as always, talk to your doctor before starting any supplement regimen to make sure it won't interfere with any medications you are taking.

Coffee

The Pros (and Cons) of a Cup of Joe

More than half of us start our morning with a cup of it. You only have to look at how many Starbucks are around (more than 12,000 worldwide) to know how popular it is.

Yet for all that coffee—and all that research that has gone along with it—researchers are undecided about whether or not it's good for your heart. Some studies say it raises cholesterol levels, and some say it lowers them. What's a coffee drinker to do?

Luckily, most of the major studies that have looked at coffee consumption and heart disease indicate that it does not raise your risk—and it may even lower it when consumed in moderation. The most notable, the Framingham Heart Study, concluded that drinking up to five cups of coffee a day may actually have lowered the risk of coronary heart disease.

The caveat is that moderation is key. Most research seems to indicate that staying under five cups a day is a good idea. Drink more, and the risks to your heart begin to rise.

What's more, the newest research on coffee and your heart seems to indicate that the way you have the coffee prepared makes a big difference in how it affects cholesterol levels. Keep reading to find out how.

The Filter Fix

In 2001, researchers at Johns Hopkins University in Baltimore reviewed more than a dozen studies that looked at the link between coffee and cholesterol. After performing the review, they noticed a surprising trend. In almost every case, the rise in cholesterol was linked to unfiltered coffee.

Though the exact reason that unfiltered coffee appears to be worse for you than filtered coffee is not completely clear, evidence seems to lean toward terpenes, oils in coffee that are mostly removed through the filtration process. Regardless of the reason, the most obvious way to avoid the risks of unfiltered coffee is to switch to filtered coffees—which most Americans drink already. Still, if you're a fan of espresso, or make your coffee with a French press or a percolator, you may want to make the switch.

How Much to Drink?

Besides how it's prepared, the other part of the coffee conundrum is how much you should drink. Researchers at Boston University polled 858 women hospitalized with a first heart attack and an equal number of healthy women on their health habits, including coffee consumption. Researchers found that compared with non–coffee drinkers, women who said they drank five to six cups of coffee a day had a 40 percent greater risk of having a heart attack, and women who drank seven to nine cups, a 70 percent greater risk. But women who drank less than five cups of coffee a day had no higher risk than women who didn't drink coffee at all.

Investigators at Kaiser Permanente Medical Center in Oakland, California, evaluated the relationship between coffee and tea intake and mortality rate—including deaths from coronary heart disease—in nearly 129,000 people. After an 8-year follow-up period, neither coffee nor tea was found to have increased the overall death rate in these people. Drinking four or more cups of coffee a day was tied to a slightly higher risk of death from heart attack, however.

Researchers at Johns Hopkins Medical Institutions in Baltimore had 100 healthy men drink varying amounts of filtered coffee: 24 ounces of regular coffee, 12 ounces of regular coffee, 24 ounces of decaffeinated coffee, or no coffee at all. After 8 weeks, the men who drank the 24 ounces of regular coffee a day experienced small increases in their total cholesterol, due to slight rises in their "bad" LDL and "good" HDL cholesterol. The researchers concluded that these small increases in LDL and HDL together "should not affect coronary heart disease risk."

In Israel, researchers analyzed coffee and tea consumption and cholesterol levels in 5,369 people. The investigators' conclusion: People who drank five or more cups of coffee a day had higher levels of total cholesterol—as much as 18 milligrams/deciliter higher—than those who abstained from coffee. The researchers also noted that the people who drank the most coffee in their study were the most likely to have negative health habits, especially smoking. "It is conceivable that the increased cholesterol levels in smokers may be confounded by coffee drinking," wrote the researchers.

Some coffee drinkers may make other lifestyle choices that may be responsible for elevating their cholesterol levels, suggests Connie Diekman, RD, director of nutrition at Washington University in St. Louis and a spokesperson for the American Dietetic Association. For example, "caffeine tends to stimulate hunger in certain people," says Diekman. "Some people may respond by eating foods that increase their cholesterol levels. But it's difficult to isolate the effect of caffeine on cholesterol and to determine whether the increases in cholesterol are caused by caffeine or by something else."

Watch the Lattes

Most people don't have to be overly anxious about their caffeine intakes, says Robert J. Nicolosi, PhD, director of the Cardiovascular Research Center at the University of Lowell in Massachusetts. "In my view, avoiding caffeine is not one of the lifestyle interventions you need to be most concerned about," says Dr. Nicolosi. While it's possible that caffeine may contribute to elevated cholesterol, he says, "the evidence is very weak at this point."

Diekman concurs. "If you enjoy coffee in moderation and it's not affecting your body—such as accelerating your heart rate—continue to drink it," she says. "But keep in mind that coffee provides no nutritional value. So make sure it's not crowding nourishing beverages (such as juice or fat-free milk) out of your diet."

What about Decaf?

You drink decaffeinated coffee, so it can't possibly affect your cholesterol. Right? Not so fast. In one study, decaffeinated coffee raised levels of "bad" LDL cholesterol, while regular, caffeinated coffee did not.

Scientists at the Lipid Research Clinic at Stanford University had 181 healthy middle-aged men drink several cups of regular, drip-filtered coffee a day. After 2 months, some of the men switched to decaf; others continued to drink regular coffee. After another 2 months, the decaf drinkers saw their LDL cholesterol increase significantly. The regular-coffee drinkers experienced no such changes in LDL. Further, the LDL cholesterol levels of the decaf drinkers were 6 percent higher than those of the regular-coffee drinkers.

The researchers' conclusion: It is not the caffeine in coffee but some other factor in the decaf that's responsible for the increase in LDL cholesterol.

Still, before you throw out all your decaffeinated coffee, keep in mind that this is just one study, and more research is necessary before a definitive conclusion can be made.

Of course, a relatively harmless morning fix can become much more harmful when it contains a generous amount of cream or half-and-half that's loaded with saturated fat—not to mention all that sugar. So it's best to drink your coffee black, or with a little fat-free or low-fat milk. Also, beware of the specialty drinks at coffee chains. Some of them are more dessert than coffee, and even the seemingly harmless ones may have more to them than meets the eye.

"Most people think that a cappuccino is 6 ounces of coffee and 2 ounces of whipped milk," says Barbie Casselman, a nutrition consultant in Toronto. "But a regular-size cappuccino is actually 2 ounces of espresso plus a cup of milk; in a large cappuccino, 12 ounces of milk. If whole milk is used, you might be consuming about 200 calories and 8 grams of fat in that 12 ounces of milk. You could eat a dessert for that!"

Heart-Healthy Indulgences

Chicory: A Coffee Substitute That Clobbers Cholesterol

In the United States, coffee is still the beverage of choice for most people. In countries like the Netherlands and Belgium, however, chicory is used as a wake-up brew, and it seems that they're onto a good thing. Research suggests that chicory is good for the heart.

One study found that chicory reduced cholesterol levels and raised the ratio of HDL to LDL in the blood of the animals tested. Evidence also shows that two substances in chicory, inulin and oligofructose, help the intestinal system by promoting the growth of good bacteria (similar to those in yogurt) and may aid in preventing osteoporosis. Early tests on animals also indicated some good results in preventing and inhibiting colon and breast cancer.

If you're interested in trying chicory, be willing to give it some time: It has a slightly bitter taste that takes some getting used to, but most people become accustomed to it after a while. Or if you'd prefer a slower transition to chicory, try New Orleans–style coffee. It has the chicory mixed in with regular coffee to enhance the flavor.

Coffee Caveats

The jury is out on whether there's an association between coffee consumption and elevated blood cholesterol. But there's less doubt, say experts, that caffeine can affect your nerves—and your bones.

"I consider caffeine to be a mind-altering drug, in the same category as nicotine and alcohol," says Dr. Nicolosi. "Some people are super-sensitive to caffeine and become hyperactive when drinking coffee." These people should consider limiting their consumption of caffeine, he says.

Caffeine may also encourage the development of osteoporosis, the bone-thinning disease that affects many women (and men) later in life, says Isadore Rosenfeld, MD, author of *Doctor, What Should I Eat?* "Caffeine steals calcium from the body by causing more of it to be excreted in the urine," says Dr. Rosenfeld. He notes, though, that "there's some research to show that drinking a glass of fat-free milk a day can offset the losses caused by coffee. So make sure you're getting plenty of calcium from milk and other sources."

Two health conditions in which some experts advise reducing or completely eliminating caffeine are heart disease and pregnancy. They recommend that people at high risk for heart attack consider drinking less coffee—under four cups a day, according to some research. And while it's not certain whether caffeine can harm a developing fetus, cautious mothers-to-be may choose to avoid caffeine during their entire pregnancies, recommends Evelyn Tribole, RD, a dietitian in Beverly Hills, California, and author of *Healthy Homestyle Cooking*.

See also Green Tea, Smoking Cessation

Cooking
Heart-Healthy Versions of Your Favorite Foods

It's one of the great ironies of life—everything that tastes good is bad for us. Fried chicken, fettuccine Alfredo, lasagna, and chili make many of our stomachs rumble. But our sensible side tells us that these foods can wreak havoc on our waistlines—and on our cholesterol levels.

But let's face it—as much as we want to eat healthier foods and look out for our heart health, sometimes replacing pasta with a salad just doesn't quite cut it. The secret, then, is to create your favorite dishes without all the fat, calories, and other heart-hurting ingredients.

Luckily for you, many of America's top dietitians, chefs, and cookbook authors know how much we like this food. And they have a number of tricks up their sleeves for transforming our favorite fattening dishes into heart-healthy helpings. They do it by replacing unhealthy ingredients with healthy ones, and even sneaking a few heart-helping ingredients into the mix. And the best part is, your taste buds will be none the wiser.

So the next time you miss meat loaf, go ahead and have it, but just make it with the heart-healthy tips below. We polled a handful of America's top dietitians and cookbook authors to come up with a list of tips for meat loaf as well as for 10 other of America's favorite foods. Start eating them this way, and chances are you won't even notice the difference in the flavor. What you probably will notice, though, is a big difference in how good you feel and how good you look. Your heart will thank you later.

Chili and Chowder

Chili con carne. The best way to bust fat and cholesterol in chili, as you can imagine, is to lose the beef and replace it with more beans. Beans are a great source of fiber and monounsaturated fat, two cholesterol-busting ingredients. But if you can't do chili without meat, try ground turkey instead of ground beef. Chances are that you won't notice the difference. And whichever meat you use, "stir-fry the meat and drain off the fat before adding it to the pot," says Wahida Karmally, RD, director of nutrition at the Irving Center for Clinical Research at Columbia-Presbyterian Medical Center in New York City and a member of the American Heart Association's nutrition committee.

Clam chowder. At first glance, creamy clam chowder seems like it's impervious to being made healthy. But it can be done: Substitute 1% milk for whole milk and fat-free evaporated milk for cream, suggests Evelyn Tribole, RD, a dietitian in Beverly Hills, California, and author of *Healthy Homestyle Cooking*. And if you usually add bacon to your chowder recipe, "use a dash of liquid smoke instead," she says.

Casseroles and Pasta Dishes

Beef stroganoff. Instead of using canned cream of mushroom soup, the traditional ingredient in this family favorite, "mix an envelope of onion-mushroom soup mix with a cup of fat-free evaporated milk and some cornstarch," says Tribole. Bring the sauce to a boil, add the beef, and serve over noodles. Then, instead of topping it off with full-fat sour cream, add a dollop of fat-free yogurt, if desired.

Lasagna. To "defat" traditional lasagna, you can choose ingredients such as lean ground beef, reduced-fat ricotta cheese, and light spaghetti sauce. But if you take an entirely different approach to lasagna, it can become a delicious vegetarian meal with a host of bold new flavors that you've never imagined. "Layer the noodles with vegetables instead of with fatty meats such as sausage," suggests Julia Della Croce, author of *The Vegetarian Table*. She suggests roasting or grilling (not frying) zucchini or eggplant, then layering the vegetables with the noodles.

Spaghetti and meatballs. Like lasagna, spaghetti is a dish that can get an injection of great flavor (and health!) with some added vegetables. Substitute a tangy blend of chopped fresh tomatoes, basil, garlic, and balsamic vinegar for the traditional meat- or sausage-filled sauce, suggests Dean Ornish, MD, president and director of the Preventive Medicine Research Institute in Sausalito, California, and author of *Dr. Dean Ornish's Program for Reversing Heart Disease*.

As for the traditional spaghetti-topper, meatballs, "try adding crumbled soy burgers—they taste just like meat," says Dr. Ornish. Or use one of the many vegetable burgers on the market.

Low-Cholesterol Cooking 101

Here are the basics of low-cholesterol cookery.

- Trim all visible fat from meat before cooking. Also, before you eat poultry, you should remove the skin.

- Bake, broil, braise, grill, boil, or steam foods, advises dietitian Marilyn Guthrie, RD, manager of health promotion at Virginia Mason Medical Center in Seattle.

- In baked goods use fat-free milk rather than whole milk. Your taste buds will never notice the difference.

- When stir-frying or sautéing foods, use nonstick cooking spray. Or you can replace each tablespoon of oil in a recipe with a teaspoon of oil plus a few tablespoons of chicken or beef broth.

More Main Dishes

Meat loaf. Using egg whites instead of whole eggs, along with very lean ground beef, will go a long way toward making meat loaf a healthier dish, says Lynn Fischer, author of *Healthy Indulgences*. To really boost the heart health of meat loaf, though, consider replacing half of the ground beef with a packaged soy mixture (available in most health food stores), she suggests. To keep the meat loaf moist, add chopped onions, celery, carrots, mushrooms, green peppers, or the whites of hard-cooked eggs. Fischer also suggests baking the meat loaf in a perforated pan; suspend the pan over a rack so that the fat can drain off.

Sauces and Stuffings

Fettuccine sauce. Few foods can clog the arteries quite like this rich pasta sauce, but even it can be made healthy. Blend fat-free cream cheese, fat-free milk, and fat-free cottage cheese in a food processor for about 4 minutes, then heat, suggests Fischer. Add ¼ cup of very lean diced ham and 1 cup of peas, if desired, she says.

   Quick and healthy gravy. To prepare a tasty make-ahead sauce for chicken, freeze chicken stock in ice cube trays, suggests Sue Chapman, executive chef at the Skylonda Fitness Retreat in Woodside, California. "When you're ready to make the sauce, melt a few cubes, then add a bit of red wine

Low-Fat Alternatives to High-Fat Ingredients

Want to make your next meal a cholesterol-busting bonanza? Cut the fat—and the cholesterol—with these heart-smart substitutes.

When You Need . . .	Use . . .
Butter, lard, or shortening	Nonstick cooking spray; olive or canola oil
Cream	Fat-free evaporated milk; fat-free milk; 1% milk
Oil or margarine	Applesauce (for muffins and quick breads)
Sour cream	Fat-free or low-fat plain yogurt; pureed 1% cottage cheese with a little lemon juice
Whipped cream	Whipped fat-free evaporated milk
Whole eggs	Egg substitute; egg whites
Whole milk	Fat-free evaporated milk; fat-free milk; 1% milk; reconstituted nonfat dry milk

and some fresh herbs such as rosemary," she says. "This sauce delivers the flavor of a traditional gravy without the fat."

Stuffing. Here is Tribole's reduced-fat version of a holiday favorite: Preheat the oven to 350°F. Sauté chopped onions, celery, and mushrooms in a nonstick skillet coated with a nonstick cooking spray. Place unseasoned cornbread stuffing in a 2-quart casserole, add the sautéed vegetables and some defatted chicken broth, then bake for 30 to 40 minutes.

Miscellaneous Goodies

French toast. Dunk your bread in egg substitute instead of whole eggs, suggests Fischer, and "fry" it in a nonstick skillet coated with a nonstick cooking spray rather than butter. You can enjoy French toast with a small amount of maple syrup, says Fischer; "just don't top it with a big hunk of butter," she advises.

Potato salad. Replace whole hard-cooked eggs with just the egg whites and whole-fat mayonnaise with the reduced-fat or fat-free variety, suggests Fischer. "The fat-free mayonnaise products available today are wonderful," she says. To boost the flavor of this salad, "try adding chopped Spanish onions, celery, dill pickles, and scallions," she says.

See also Eggs, Fat-Free Milk, Fish, Lean Meat, Mediterranean Diet, Vegetables

Dark Leafy Greens
The Darker, the Better

Call it the "American paradox"—give us a category of food, even a seemingly healthy category like leafy vegetables, and somehow we'll gravitate toward the least healthy one of the bunch.

Unfortunately, such is the case with salad greens. For decades, America's favorite salad starter has been iceberg lettuce. And while iceberg is not necessarily an unhealthy choice, it literally "pales" in comparison to its darker, healthier cousins such as kale, Swiss chard, beet greens, mustard greens, turnip greens, and spinach.

Luckily, it's not that difficult to select healthier greens in the produce aisle of your grocery store. You may have noticed lately that a lot of health advisories have tacked the words "brightly colored" to their recommendation to eat more fruits and vegetables, and there's a simple reason for this. "The darker the color, the more nutrients and antioxidant compounds the fruits or vegetables will have," says Christopher Gardner, PhD, of the Stanford Prevention Research Center at Stanford University Medical Center.

How Greens Help the Heart

This "darker is better" concept definitely applies to leafy green vegetables. In fact, few foods in our diet deliver more nutrients with fewer calories than greens do. Add greens to your diet, and you'll get a treasure trove of valuable nutrients—magnesium, iron, calcium, folate, vitamin C, vitamin B_6, plus all the flavonoids that offer additional heart protection.

When it comes to heart health, all of these nutrients are helpful. But it's the B vitamins (B_6 and folate) that are of specific interest. These appear to regulate a compound called homocysteine in the body and keep its levels in check. In the renowned Framingham Heart Study in Massachusetts, 43 percent of men and 34 percent of women with the most-clogged arteries had high levels of homocysteine in their blood.

Getting More Greens

Replacing iceberg lettuce with spinach in salads is a great way to get more greens, but you should look for other places to replace lettuce with healthier spinach, such as on sandwiches or burgers. Greens are also quite easy to cook as a side dish for any meal and will retain most of their nutrients if prepared properly. Here are some tips for doing just that:

• Remove stems. Though the leaves are tender, most greens have tough, chewy stems. It's best to remove these completely prior to cooking.

• Rinse thoroughly. The textured leaves of many greens can trap a lot of dirt and grit. Wash them several times to get them clean.

• Cut ribbons. Many greens are quite thick and have large leaves. To help them cook more quickly, as well as to make them easier to eat, cut the leaves into small ribbons before cooking.

• Wilt tender greens. For the most tender greens, like beet greens or spinach, you can wilt them simply by pouring boiling water over them and draining them immediately. Or just stir them together with already warm ingredients like pasta or potatoes.

• Boil or braise tougher greens. Some of the tougher greens, like turnips or collards, may require boiling or braising. Boiling requires submerging the greens in boiling water for 15 to 20 minutes. You can use bacon or ham hock for added flavor, if desired. Braising is done for a similar amount of time but with less liquid over a lower heat and using a tight-fitting lid. Chicken stock, vegetable stock, olive oil, and wine are often used for braising to add flavor to the greens.

Eggs

Playing the Shell Game with Your Heart

A lot of foods seem to send mixed messages when put under the microscope for scientific study. But few have gone back and forth quite as much as eggs. Media reports on eggs have switched sides so many times that it has become almost comical. Ask most people whether eggs are healthy or not, and they might tell you that it depends on which way the wind is blowing that day.

The fact is, researchers are learning new things about foods all the time. And because the media is often quick to react, sometimes judgments about foods are made before all the information is in. Eggs have definitely been a victim of that.

To cut through the confusion, we'll try to provide an overview of eggs: the good, the bad, and the ugly. But let's start with the best: Most people can still eat eggs as part of a heart-healthy diet.

Eggs Aren't All Bad

Eggs definitely have their good points. One large egg is brimming with vitamins E and B_{12}, folate, riboflavin, phosphorus, and iron and has less than 2 grams of saturated fat.

Eggs also are a rich source of protein. "Eggs are the best-quality, least expensive protein we can eat," says Wanda Howell, PhD, RD, distinguished professor of nutritional sciences at the University of Arizona in Tucson. For elderly folks on fixed incomes, this can be particularly important, as they provide the protein this population needs at a price they can afford.

Packed with Cholesterol

Unfortunately, many people—including the elderly—tend to steer clear of eggs, despite all this protein. And that's because egg yolks are the richest source of cholesterol in our diets. The yolk of one average egg contains 213 milligrams of dietary cholesterol—more than two-thirds of the daily limit of 300 milligrams recommended by the American Heart Association (AHA).

The AHA says that healthy adults can eat up to four whole eggs per week but advises people with elevated cholesterol to limit themselves to one whole egg a week. "Because eggs—or more specifically, egg yolks—are a concentrated source of dietary cholesterol, you shouldn't overdo them," says Alicia Moag-Stahlberg, RD, a dietitian with Action for Healthy Kids, a nonprofit

Love to Bake? Lose the Yolks!

You don't have to forgo baking—or eating—your favorite cakes, cookies, and muffins because you're cutting back on eggs. Here's how to bake yolk-free treats.

Baking with egg whites. Not using egg yolks won't significantly affect the texture of baked goods, says Evelyn Tribole, RD, a dietitian in Beverly Hills, California, and author of *Healthy Homestyle Cooking*. "Most likely, you won't notice the difference," she says. She recommends substituting two beaten egg whites for each whole egg.

If you're baking a product that calls for three or four whole eggs, however, substituting that many egg whites may create too much liquid. In that case, you may want to use an egg substitute.

Baking with egg substitute. Some experts suggest replacing each whole egg with ¼ cup of egg substitute, but you can use more or less of this product to suit your taste.

organization located in Chicago, whose mission is to improve children's nutrition and physical activity.

However, don't be misled into avoiding eggs entirely. Though eggs do seem to raise cholesterol in the body somewhat, the newest research indicates that the way in which eggs raise cholesterol may be less of a concern than with some other foods.

In a study of middle-aged and elderly people presented by the University of Connecticut in 2006, researchers found that eating three large eggs per day did tend to elevate levels of "bad" LDL cholesterol. But it also raised levels of "good" HDL cholesterol, to the point where the effect was essentially neutral.

In addition, as our understanding of cholesterol is becoming more sophisticated, so is our understanding of eggs. Cholesterol isn't just LDL and HDL: There are lipoproteins in both categories that come in varying sizes. In both LDL and HDL, the larger particles are better. Larger low-density lipoproteins are less likely to embed themselves in the arterial walls and lead to atherosclerosis. And larger high-density lipoproteins are more likely to grab other lipoproteins and other heart-hurting particles and shuttle them out of the body.

Keeping this in mind, the researchers at the University of Connecticut found that the cholesterol from eggs almost always manifests itself in the body as larger particles. That means the LDL produced from eggs is less likely to cause heart disease.

A Strong Response to Eggs

Despite these promising findings, the AHA's rule of "four eggs per week" is still a good one to go by. And for up to 30 to 40 percent of the population, it's particularly important. Almost this many people might be "responders" to eggs, which means that eggs will make their cholesterol spike much higher than the rest of the population's.

In one study, 25 people were asked to eat 12 eggs a week for 6 weeks. In 23 of the participants, cholesterol levels stayed the same. In the other two, LDL cholesterol rose by 25 percent. That translates into a 50 percent increase in the estimated risk of a heart attack.

There's no way to know if you'll be a responder, so study author Nancy Lewis, PhD, RD, a nutritionist at the University of Nebraska in Lincoln, recommends that you have your cholesterol checked a month or so after adding eggs to your diet. If your numbers have spiked upward, switch back to egg substitutes. (If you have diabetes, you should avoid eggs completely, according to a Harvard study.)

Considering all these findings, the key advice here is to not get hung up on eggs and disregard the rest of your diet. While cutting back on dietary cholesterol can often help lower your blood cholesterol, "reducing your intake of total and saturated fat will help even more," says Dr. Howell.

Breaking Free of the Yolk

As mentioned, only egg yolks contain dietary cholesterol, which means you can eat as many egg whites as you wish. Doesn't sound like much of a treat, you say? Get creative! Here are some ideas to get you started.

Heart-Healthy Indulgences

Omega-3–Enriched Eggs: For More Heart-Friendly Omelets

You probably never thought you'd see the day when eggs were promoted for their benefits. As unlikely as it seemed, however, that day has arrived.

Scientists have known for some time that omega-3 fatty acids, found primarily in fish, benefit heart health. But omega-3s can now be found in some eggs, since egg producers are feeding hens flaxseed meal, fish meal, or marine algae, all of which contain the fatty acids.

The amount of omega-3s that you'll get depends on the product you buy. Choice Eggs, for example, contain 350 milligrams of omega-3 fats per egg.

The omega-3s help you by protecting your heart and improving your mood. Even people with diabetes or high cholesterol can eat up to four eggs a week, and most healthy people can eat up to an egg a day, or seven a week.

Start with the frittata on page 56, an "Italian omelet." By combining egg whites and whole eggs, you can reduce fat and cholesterol without compromising taste.

• It's possible for you to create an appetizing breakfast without using whole eggs. "You don't have to sacrifice flavor," says Evelyn Tribole, RD, a dietitian in Beverly Hills, California, and author of *Healthy Homestyle Cooking.* "Try making French toast with egg whites and fat-free milk. Or make egg-white omelets stuffed with bell peppers, mushrooms, and onions. Chopped green chile peppers work well, too." But don't sauté all of those vegetables in butter. Use a nonstick cooking spray instead.

• Make cholesterol-free *huevos rancheros*, suggests Marvin Moser, MD, clinical professor of medicine at Yale University School of Medicine and author of *Week by Week to a Strong Heart.* Simply fold scrambled egg whites into a taco or tortilla, then top the eggs with spicy salsa.

Try This Tasty Impostor

Yearning for a plate of steaming scrambled eggs? You can indulge your craving with egg substitutes. These products consist primarily of egg whites, with other ingredients—including fat-free milk, food coloring, vegetable oil, and vitamins—added to mimic the taste and texture of real eggs and to boost nutritional value. Most egg substitutes contain zero cholesterol and 1 to 4 grams of fat per serving.

Use egg substitute as you would egg whites or even whole eggs. You can make a tasty omelet by adding chopped onions, mushrooms, peppers, and reduced-fat or fat-free cheese to egg substitute, for example. Or you can mix this product with flavored bread crumbs to batter-coat baked chicken (without the skin).

There's one advantage of using egg substitute over egg whites explains, Tribole: It's yellow, so it looks like the real thing. "If you like scrambled eggs and you're really into eye appeal, use egg substitute," she says. And with more and more restaurants offering omelets and scrambled eggs made with egg substitute, it's not difficult to follow your program away from home.

Two Ways to Have Your Eggs and Eat Them, Too

Sometimes only real eggs will do. If you have elevated cholesterol, most doctors agree that it's smart to stick to the AHA's guidelines and limit yourself to one whole egg per week. Within that guideline, if egg substitute or egg whites just aren't for you, it's possible to occasionally eat whole eggs as part of an overall low-fat, low-cholesterol diet. Try these suggestions.

• Instead of large or jumbo-size eggs, go for the small or medium-size ones. By simply downsizing, you can cut out some extra cholesterol.

Spinach and Mushroom Frittata

Makes 4 servings

- ½ cup chopped onion
- 4 ounces mushrooms, sliced
- 5 ounces frozen chopped spinach, thawed and squeezed dry
- 4 omega-3-enriched eggs
- 6 egg whites
- 2 teaspoons water
- 1 tablespoon chopped fresh thyme
- 1 tablespoon chopped fresh oregano or marjoram
- ½ teaspoon salt
  Pinch of ground black pepper

Coat a large ovenproof nonstick skillet with cooking spray. Warm the skillet over medium heat until hot. Add the onion and mushrooms and cook, stirring frequently, for 4 minutes, or until the mushrooms begin to release their liquid.

Add the spinach and cook, stirring frequently, for 5 minutes, or until most of the liquid has evaporated.

Meanwhile, in a medium bowl, beat together the eggs, egg whites, water, thyme, oregano or marjoram, salt, and pepper. Add to the skillet and swirl to evenly distribute the mixture. Cook over medium heat for 5 minutes, gently lifting the egg mixture from the sides of the skillet with a spatula as it becomes set. Cook until the eggs are set on the bottom but still moist on the top. Remove from the heat.

Wrap the handle of the skillet with 2 layers of heavy foil. Broil 4" from the heat for 1 minute, or until the top is golden.

Use a spatula to loosen the frittata and slide it onto a serving plate. Cut into wedges and serve.

Per serving: 123 calories, 5.2 g fat (39% of calories), 13.1 g protein, 5.7 g carbohydrates, 213 mg cholesterol, 0.7 g dietary fiber, 434 mg sodium

• Never scramble or fry eggs in bacon grease or butter. Both are loaded with saturated fat. Instead, prepare them in a nonstick skillet coated with cooking spray. Or try eating eggs hard-cooked or poached, suggests Dr. Howell.

Exercise

Sweat Your Way to More "Good" Cholesterol

When it comes to our heart health, we tend to get bogged down in the small stuff. And while these little things are undoubtedly important, experts will tell you time and again that your heart health comes down to two basic strategies: maintaining a healthy weight and getting more exercise.

The federal government understands this. That's why in 2005 they upgraded—no, overhauled—their exercise guidelines. The old recommendations called for 30 minutes of exercise every day. Now, that's the absolute minimum. If you want to maintain weight and prevent weight gain, you should exercise for 60 minutes a day. And if you'd like to lose weight or maintain weight loss after previously losing weight, the recommendation is 60 to 90 minutes. That's quite a jump!

But don't worry. Adding an hour of activity to your day is a lot easier than you might think. Read on to see how do it—and why you'll want to in the first place.

The Dream Team

According to scientific evidence, exercise helps boost levels of "good" HDL cholesterol, which helps whisk "bad" LDL cholesterol out of the body. "It is thought that exercise's ability to reduce the risk of heart disease comes mostly from its ability to increase HDL cholesterol," says James Rippe, MD, director of the Center for Clinical and Lifestyle Research at Tufts University School of Medicine in Boston and coauthor of *Dr. James Rippe's Complete Book of Fitness Walking.*

In a recent study at Duke University in Durham, North Carolina, researchers looked at the effect of exercise on a group of 182 sedentary and overweight men and women at risk of developing diabetes or heart disease. They divided them into three groups—low-, moderate-, or high-intensity training—and then put them through 8 months of exercise training.

The results were significant. All three groups experienced a drop in triglycerides, and the amount of that reduction correlated with the intensity of the exercise program. (The high-intensity group noticed the greatest benefit, and the low-intensity group noticed the least.) In addition, the exercisers experienced a boost in "good" HDL cholesterol and an overall improvement in lipoprotein size. (The newest research has shown that larger cholesterol lipoproteins are advantageous compared to smaller ones.)

The researchers found that the exercisers in the high-intensity group sustained some additional benefit in their triglyceride levels even 14 days after the end of their training. Those in the other two groups did not see this benefit. But the best news is that most of the people didn't want to stop exercising after their 8 months of training. "When we asked the participants to stop their exercise program, there were a lot of grumpy people," says Johanna Johnson, a clinical research coordinator in the School of Medicine at Duke

---

How to Find Your Target Heart Rate

While you work out, periodically check your pulse to be sure you're in your target heart range, suggests James Rippe, MD, director of the Center for Clinical and Lifestyle Research at Tufts University School of Medicine in Boston and coauthor of *Dr. James Rippe's Complete Book of Fitness Walking.*

To get the low number for your range, subtract your age from 220, then multiply that figure by 0.6. To get the high number for your range, subtract your age from 220, then multiply by 0.85.

If you're 52 years old, for example, you'd subtract 52 from 220, which equals 168. Multiply 168 by 0.6, which equals 100.8 (low number for your range). Multiply 168 by 0.85, which equals 142.8 (high number for your range). Your heart rate should remain between 101 and 142 as you exercise.

Some experts suggest that there's a simpler way to gauge whether you're overextending yourself. "If you can't carry on a conversation during exercise, you're overdoing it," says John McDougall, MD, founder of the McDougall Program and McDougall Health Center in Santa Rosa, California, and author of *McDougall's Heart Medicine.*

University. "After 8 to 9 months of exercise, it had become a part of their routine."

As for the effect on triglycerides, exercise appears to trigger a chain of physiological events that increase the efficiency of an enzyme called lipoprotein lipase, says Michael Miller, MD, director of preventive cardiology at the University of Maryland Medical Center in Baltimore. This enzyme attacks triglycerides. "As lipoprotein lipase breaks down triglyceride-rich particles, it also produces substances that help make HDL," explains Dr. Miller. So people who exercise tend to make more HDL and have lower triglyceride levels, he says.

Researchers at the University of Hawaii at Manoa in Honolulu analyzed the effect of exercise on HDL levels in 10 separate studies involving about 700 people. The researchers found that for each 6.2 miles per week that a person jogged, HDL climbed 3 milligrams/deciliter in both men and women.

Regular exercise also helps you lose weight, which can further improve your cholesterol profile. One well-known study determined that for every 8 pounds a person sheds, HDL rises about 3 points. And for every 8 pounds gained, HDL declines about 2 points.

Choose Your Own Adventure

The good news is, you don't have to become a marathon runner to raise your HDL and slash your risk of heart disease. In fact, you may want to avoid doing that. "It appears that too much activity might be counterproductive, especially when it comes to running marathons, as new studies suggest that there may be more rapid development of calcium in the heart vessels leading to premature heart disease," says Dr. Miller.

Instead, Dr. Miller advocates a moderate program to reap the heart-healthy benefits of exercise. It's best to start with a 5- to 10-minute warmup period, followed by more brisk activity for 20 to 30 minutes, and then another 5- to 10-minute cooldown, he says. "A person with high cholesterol and/or other heart disease risk factors may need further testing if he or she has not been active and wishes to engage in aerobic activities."

Get moving, though, and the results can be significant. "It seems that if you burn at least 1,200 calories per week, you'll see increases in HDL cholesterol," says Dr. Miller. "Overall, aerobic activity can lower triglycerides 20 to 40 percent and raise HDL 10 to 20 percent."

Knock Down Cholesterol with Exercise *and* Diet

While exercise has been proven to lower the risk of coronary heart disease, exercise combined with a low-fat diet can pack an even stronger punch.

Researchers at Stanford University School of Medicine had one group of moderately overweight people follow a low-fat, low-cholesterol diet. A second group followed the same diet but also exercised three times a week. After a year, the exercisers raised their HDL levels by an average of 13 percent. By contrast, the diet-only group raised their HDL just 2 percent.

Nine Heart-Healthy Fitness Tips

There's no denying the proven benefits of regular exercise, from a healthier heart to a better shape. So don your workout clothes and get moving! These tips can help make it easier.

- Put your goals in writing. You're more likely to stick to an exercise program if you know what you want to accomplish and write it down, says exercise physiologist Peter Snell, PhD, assistant professor of internal medi-

---

Can Pumping Iron Help Pump Up HDL?

Most health professionals recommend aerobic exercise to help raise "good" HDL cholesterol and protect against heart disease. But there's some preliminary evidence that a nonaerobic activity—weight training—may help lower cholesterol as well.

Researchers at the Department of Veteran Affairs Medical Center and the University of Arizona, both in Tucson, enrolled 46 women in a weight-training program. These women pumped iron for an hour three times a week. Another group of women acted as a control group, sticking to their normal exercise habits.

After 5 months, the women involved in weight training saw their total cholesterol drop from 184 to 171 milligrams/deciliter (mg/dl). More significantly, their LDL cholesterol plummeted by 12 percent, from 116 to 102 mg/dl, with no significant effect on their HDL levels.

If you're not interested in becoming the next world's strongest man (or woman), you're in luck. You can combine aerobic and nonaerobic exercise in simple ways to get the benefits of both. "Both appear to be beneficial, and aerobic activity coupled with muscle toning improves the efficiency of oxygen delivery to muscles and is additive toward heart protection," says Michael Miller, MD, director of preventive cardiology at the University of Maryland Medical Center in Baltimore. "So carrying a light weight while walking briskly appears to provide added advantage."

cine at the University of Texas Southwestern Medical Center at Dallas. "Start keeping a workout log," he suggests. "The log will be a record of what you've accomplished and will help keep you on track."

• Find a workout you enjoy. From fencing to inline skating to yoga, there's a wealth of fitness options that you may not have considered. So explore the alternatives. "When you're having fun being physically active, you're much more likely to keep going, week after week and month after month," says Darlene A. Sedlock, PhD, associate professor of kinesiology at Purdue University in West Lafayette, Indiana.

• Go at your own pace. "Don't adhere to the adage 'No pain, no gain,'" says Dr. Sedlock. "Do what you're capable of doing. You'll find that exercise becomes easier and easier."

• Schedule a "happy hour" for exercise. "If you commit to working out at a particular time and place, you'll have a greater chance of meeting your goals," says Dr. Rippe. Try taking an aerobics class during your lunch hour, for example, or enjoy a brisk walk after dinner.

• Work out with a friend who's at a similar fitness level, suggests Dr. Snell.

• Vary your activities—walk on Monday, cycle on Wednesday, play a round of golf on Sunday, and so forth. If you walk regularly, "give yourself a change of scenery by varying your walking route," advises Dr. Rippe. Should you grow weary of your regular Tuesday-night step class, drop in on that Friday-night disco aerobics class that you've been meaning to try.

• If you exercise outdoors, adapt to the weather. "In cold weather, dress in layers that you can remove as your body heats up," says Dr. Rippe. In warm weather, he says, wear loose clothing and drink lots of water before and during your workout. In stormy weather, try walking on an indoor track at the health club or at the mall.

• Add more activity to your day. At work, you might forgo your midmorning coffee break and go on a short walk instead. Or resolve to take the stairs instead of the elevator at least once a day.

• Reward yourself for meeting your exercise goals. Buy a new shade of lipstick or a new tie. Splurge on some new workout gear. "Even a hot bath can be a reward," says Dr. Rippe.

See also Walking

Fat-Free Milk

The Skinny on Skim

Let's face it—with all the new research about the effects of saturated fat on your heart, milk may not seem like a food that does a body good. When it comes to this artery-clogging fat, whole milk is one of the richest sources of it in our diets. A cup of whole milk is 49 percent fat, most of it saturated. It also packs a whopping punch of 33 milligrams of cholesterol and 150 calories. And despite its name, 2% milk doesn't fare much better—it is still 34 percent fat.

But the news about milk isn't all bad. After all, it's a rich source of calcium, which, aside from building bones, is a key agent in lowering cholesterol. It's a great source of protein, as well as vitamin D, which also promotes bone health; potassium, which offers additional heart help; and riboflavin. The nutrients in milk have been connected to the prevention of high blood pressure, stroke, osteoporosis, and even cancer. The only problem is all that pesky fat!

Enter fat-free milk, also known as nonfat or skim milk. Fat-free milk has been stripped of almost all the saturated fat of its whole and 2% counterparts, but it retains all the nutrients. The result is a drink with healthful benefits—and not much else. One cup of fat-free milk has 0.4 gram of fat, 4 milligrams of cholesterol, and 85 calories. And, as you'll see below, making the switch to skim can have a dramatic effect on your cholesterol levels as well as your overall heart health.

If you've shunned fat-free milk in the past, you'll want to give it another try. Milk producers have come a long way since the early days of the thin, gray, and watery stuff. Now it's creamy, flavorful, and difficult to distinguish from whole milk. Give it a few weeks, and you'll wonder why you ever complained about the difference in taste.

In addition, when you prepare your meals with fat-free milk instead of whole, you'll really be hard-pressed to notice the difference. The result is that you can still prepare all your favorite dishes without sacrificing any flavor—just fat!

Feelin' Good with Fat-Free

A number of studies have compared the effects of whole milk with those of fat-free milk on blood cholesterol. Here's what these studies have found.

Researchers at the University of Minnesota in Minneapolis and other institutions put eight healthy men on a low-fat diet that followed the guidelines of the American Heart Association. For 6 weeks of a 3-month-long study, the men drank 2 to 4 cups of whole milk per day. For the other 6 weeks, they drank an equal amount of fat-free milk. The men's total cholesterol was 7 percent lower, and their "bad" LDL cholesterol was 11 percent lower, on the skim-milk diet than on the whole-milk plan.

These researchers noted that for every 1 percent reduction in total cholesterol, the risk of coronary heart disease drops about 2 percent. Consequently, these experts proposed, healthy men with normal blood cholesterol who drink 2 to 4 cups of whole milk a day could slash their risk of coronary heart disease by about 14 percent if they switched from whole milk to fat-free.

Researchers at Kansas State University in Manhattan and Pennsylvania State University in University Park had 64 people supplement their diets with a quart of fat-free milk a day. After 2 months, people who began the study with total cholesterol of 190 milligrams/deciliter or above saw their total cholesterol decline 6.6 percent and their triglyceride levels drop almost 12 percent. The blood pressure of these men and women dropped as well, perhaps due to the calcium and potassium content of the fat-free milk.

Why Low-Fat Doesn't Quite Cut It

Using a couple of teaspoons of low-fat milk a day won't hurt you, say experts. But if every day you gulp down a couple of glasses of low-fat milk, which contains either 1 or 2 percent milk fat, you're not trimming as much fat from your diet as you may think.

At first glance, "2%" and "1%" sound pretty promising. But once water is eliminated from the calculations, 2% milk contains 20 percent fat by weight. What's more, 2% milk gets 34 percent of its calories from fat, while only 5 percent of the calories in fat-free milk come from fat.

Still not convinced? Here's one more calculation that may help you make the switch to fat-free. If you drink two glasses of 1% milk every day for a year, you're swallowing 4 pounds of fat. Drinking the same amount of fat-free milk, on the other hand, provides less than one-tenth of a pound of fat.

Fake Out Your Taste Buds

These tips can make the transition from whole or low-fat milk to fat-free milk practically painless.

• Drink fat-free milk from a frosted mug. For some reason, lowering the temperature enhances the taste.

• Don't feel you have to switch to fat-free milk right away. If you need to wean yourself off the heavy stuff, try this approach: Drink 2% milk for about a month, then switch to 1%, and finally to skim.

• Many people find it difficult to use fat-free milk on breakfast cereals, says Janet Lepke-Harris, RD, a dietitian in Charlotte, North Carolina, and a spokesperson for the American Dietetic Association. "So if you want to use 1% milk instead of fat-free on your cereal, it's no big deal," she says. (Consider making the switch to fat-free milk somewhere down the road, though.)

• If you've always used half-and-half or straight cream in your coffee, "try mixing 2 teaspoons of a liquid nondairy creamer and 2 teaspoons of 1% milk," says Marilyn Cerino, RD, nutrition consultant at the Benjamin Franklin Center for Health of Pennsylvania Hospital in Philadelphia. "This substitute looks and tastes rich."

• Love bathing your vegetables in a white cream sauce? "Mix a teaspoon each of margarine and flour, then heat for 2 minutes, slowly whisking in fat-free milk," suggests Cerino. "It makes a delicious sauce."

• If you're yearning for a rich, creamy milk shake, whip up a banana health shake, suggests Evelyn Tribole, RD, a dietitian in Beverly Hills, California, and author of *Healthy Homestyle Cooking*. Blend one ripe banana, ¼ cup of nonfat dry milk, ½ cup of orange juice, 1 teaspoon of vanilla, a dash of nutmeg, and five ice cubes until creamy. "In about a minute, you'll have made a delicious, refreshing drink containing only a trace amount of fat," says Tribole.

See also Calcium

Fiber

The Old Heart-Health Standby

Lots of fad foods have come and gone, but when it comes to your heart health, one piece of advice has remained constant—eat more fiber.

Unfortunately, thanks in large part to television commercials, most of us think of fiber as that unpleasant powder you mix with water to, you know, unbind yourself.

But in foods, fiber is a much more complicated nutrient. One kind of fiber that's used in laxatives and found in abundance in whole grains, fruits, vegetables, and cereals is known as insoluble fiber. It helps keep you regular by, shall we say, clearing out your system.

The other kind, soluble fiber, seems to do a similar thing in the blood—it flushes out cholesterol. Soluble fiber—such as pectin and guar gum, to name two kinds—is found in foods like apples, peas, oat bran, dried beans, barley, and psyllium-containing breakfast cereals. This type of fiber seems to play a key role in lowering cholesterol levels.

"I consider soluble fiber to be nature's most powerful cholesterol-lowering agent," says Ann G. Kulze, MD, founder and CEO of Just Wellness, a wellness consulting firm in Mt. Pleasant, South Carolina, and the author of *Dr. Ann's 10-Step Diet*. "Ingested soluble fiber combines with water in the GI tract and forms a gelatinous-like substance that 'sponges' up cholesterol and prevents its absorption."

Recently, new research seems to indicate that some types of soluble fiber may have more cholesterol-lowering power than others. "Both oats and barley contain a special type of soluble fiber known as beta-glucan," says Dr. Kulze. "The studies supporting beta-glucan's ability to lower cholesterol are so solid that the FDA allows foods containing 0.75 gram or more of beta-glucan per serving to carry a qualified health claim for reducing cholesterol."

Regardless of the type of fiber, scientists believe that eating a fiber-rich diet may help reduce the risk of developing colon cancer, diabetes, and other ailments as well as heart disease. All in all, good reasons to munch something that crunches—and that doesn't mean chips.

The Benefits of Bulk

Scientists have conducted numerous studies of fiber's power to stomp cholesterol. In one study, researchers at the University of Kentucky College of Medicine in Lexington divided 146 people with moderately elevated cholesterol into three groups. The first group ate their usual diets. The second group followed a low-fat diet that contained 15 grams (about ½ ounce) of fiber. The third group consumed a low-fat diet packed with 25 grams of fiber. After a year, the low-fat, high-fiber group's total cholesterol had fallen 13 percent, compared with a 9 percent drop in cholesterol for the low-fat group, and a 7 percent decrease in the folks who ate their usual diets.

In another study, researchers at Stanford University School of Medicine had 16 people consume 15 grams of soluble fiber (including pectin and psyllium) a day. These folks' total cholesterol fell 8.3 percent, and their "bad" LDL cholesterol dropped 12.4 percent, in just 1 month.

There's evidence that adding soluble fiber to a diet already low in fat can further slam cholesterol. Researchers from the United States, Canada, and Switzerland had 43 people with high cholesterol follow either a low-fat, high-soluble-fiber diet or a low-fat, high-insoluble-fiber diet for 4 months. Then the group that had followed the soluble-fiber plan consumed the diet high in insoluble fiber, and vice versa, for another 4 months. The study participants' total and LDL cholesterol levels were 5 percent lower when they consumed the diet rich in soluble fiber than when they followed the plan high in insoluble fiber.

More recently, researchers at the University of Massachusetts Medical School in Worcester may have discovered another way that fiber helps prevent heart disease—by lowering blood levels of C-reactive protein (CRP), a risk factor for future heart disease.

In this study of 524 healthy adults, the researchers measured the participants' CRP levels five times over the course of the year. They also collected information about the participants' exercise and diet habits, among other health factors. What they found was that the higher the participants' intake of fiber was, the lower the CRP levels were. And it didn't take a lot to make a difference—those who ate the most fiber in the study consumed around 22 grams a day, which is just within the recommended daily intake of 20 to 35 grams of fiber a day.

Best Food Sources of Fiber

Want to clamp down on high cholesterol? Chomp into the following foods—they're high in soluble fiber, the kind that helps lower blood cholesterol levels. Many of these foods also supply insoluble fiber, which offers other health benefits.

Food	Total Fiber (g)	Soluble Fiber (g)
All-Bran cereal (1/3 cup)	8.6	1.4
Apple, with skin (1 small)	2.8	1
Barley, raw (2 Tbsp)	3	0.9
Blackberries (3/4 cup)	3.7	1.1
Blueberries (3/4 cup)	1.4	0.3
Brussels sprouts (1 cup)	5	2.6
Carrot, raw (1)	2.3	1.1
Chickpeas (1/2 cup)	4.3	1.3
Corn bran, raw (2 Tbsp)	7.7	0.1
Figs, dried (3)	4.6	2.2
Grapefruit, pink (1)	1.4	0.3
Kidney beans, cooked (1/2 cup)	6.9	2.8
Lentils, boiled (1/2 cup)	5.2	0.6
Lima beans, canned (1/2 cup)	4.3	1.1
Oat bran, dry (1/3 cup)	4	2
Okra (1 cup)	7.3	2.9
Orange (1 small)	2.9	1.8
Pear (1 small)	2.9	1.1
Peas, frozen, cooked (1/2 cup)	4.3	1.3
Pinto beans, cooked (1/2 cup)	5.9	1.9
Plums, red, with skin (2 medium)	2.4	1.1
Potato, baked (1)	5	1.2
Pumpernickel bread (1 slice)	2.7	1.2
Raisins, seedless (1/2 cup)	1.6	0.8
Spaghetti, whole wheat, cooked (1 cup)	5.4	1.2
Spinach, boiled (1/2 cup)	1.6	0.5
Sweet potato, baked (1)	2.7	1.2
Turnips, cooked (1/2 cup)	4.8	1.7
Wheat germ, toasted (1/4 cup)	5.2	0.8
White/navy beans, cooked (1/2 cup)	6.5	2.2

How to Fill Up on Fiber

The University of Massachusetts study mentioned above proves an important point. When it comes to fiber, most of us don't get enough. "Americans consume about 12 grams of fiber (less than ½ ounce) a day," says Alicia Moag-Stahlberg, RD, a dietitian with Action for Healthy Kids, a nonprofit organization located in Chicago, whose mission is to improve children's nutrition and physical activity. "We should be eating about 25 to 30 grams (about an ounce) per day." Fortunately, it's easy to fiber up your diet. The following tips can help.

• Be sure to eat the skins of fruits and vegetables (such as apples and potatoes) as well as fruits with edible seeds, such as figs and blueberries.

The Coronary Artery Risk Development in Young Adults (CARDIA) Study, a multicenter study that examined heart disease risk factors in young men and women over a period of 10 years, showed that young adults who ate at least 21 grams of fiber a day gained 8 pounds less than people who ate the same number of calories but less than 12 grams of fiber. Since weight control also helps control cholesterol, that doubles the benefits of fiber.

• Try to get your fiber from foods rather than from fiber supplements, recommends Moag-Stahlberg. Researchers at the Northwest Lipid Research Clinic in Seattle evaluated the cholesterol-lowering effects of a dietary supplement of water-soluble fibers (guar gum and pectin) and mostly non-water-soluble fibers (soy fiber, pea fiber, and corn bran) in people with mild to moderate high cholesterol. They were randomly assigned to receive 20 grams of the fiber supplement or a placebo (an inactive substance) daily for 15 weeks. After that period, all of the participants received the fiber supplement for an additional 36 weeks.

Decreases in LDL cholesterol levels, total cholesterol levels, and LDL-to-HDL ratio were greater in the fiber group. Researchers say that the fiber supplement provided significant and sustained reductions in LDL without reducing "good" HDL and had the added bonus of not increasing triglycerides (another blood fat) over the treatment period.

However, relying on supplements as your sole source of fiber isn't ideal. The supplements lack other nutrients found in fiber-rich foods, says Moag-Stahlberg. "Fruits and vegetables contain antioxidant vitamins, for example, which may help prevent heart disease and cancer."

• Don't consume a day's worth of fiber in one sitting, advises Susan Kleiner, PhD, RD, a nutritionist in Seattle and author of *The High-Performance Cookbook*. "Eat high-fiber foods throughout the day," she advises. "Don't depend on a high-fiber cereal whose manufacturer claims that you can get all of your fiber in one bowl."

• Drink 8 to 10 glasses of water a day. Fiber absorbs fluid as it passes through the body, and not drinking enough water can lead to constipation.

• To minimize gas and bloating—common side effects of consuming more fiber—add fiber-rich foods to your diet slowly.

• Don't gobble fiber to compensate for eating high-fat foods. As Dean Ornish, MD, president and director of the Preventive Medicine Research Institute in Sausalito, California, says in *Dr. Dean Ornish's Program for Reversing Heart Disease*, "A bowl of (oatmeal) is an ideal breakfast, but it won't undo the effects of a ham-and-cheese omelet on the side."

See also Beans, Fruit, Oats, Pectin, Vegetables, Vegetarian Diet, Whole Grains

Fish

At Long Last, A Heart-Healthy Meal

Look up and down the list of heart-healthy, cholesterol-busting foods, and you'll probably notice that most of them have one thing in common: They're plants.

And that's great! Hey, we like salad as much as anyone else. But every once in a while, we crave something to fulfill our carnivorous side. Can this be done without compromising our heart health?

Luckily, the answer is yes. And the best choice you can make to satisfy your meat craving while still making your heart happy is fish.

The problem with most meats, particularly beef and pork, is that they're loaded with saturated fats. "The saturated fats are dangerous because they increase the blood levels of LDL ('bad' cholesterol) and promote its oxidation, which all leads to atherosclerotic heart disease," says Ralph Felder, MD, PhD, section chief for cardiovascular nutrition at the Good Samaritan Medical Center in Phoenix and author of *The Bonus Years Diet*. And while it's okay to eat beef and pork every once in a while, it's best to balance them out in your diet with some healthier fats.

That's where fish comes in. Fish is low in saturated fats and high in a form of polyunsaturated fat that you've probably heard of: omega-3 fatty acids. The name isn't particularly catchy—until you realize all the great things that omega-3s can do for your heart.

"Omega-3 fats are 'essential fats' that play a critical role in cardiovascular health," says Ann G. Kulze, MD, founder and CEO of Just Wellness, a wellness consulting firm in Mt. Pleasant, South Carolina, and the author of *Dr. Ann's 10-Step Diet*. "They do not specifically lower cholesterol, but they have a number of other benefits, including decreasing triglycerides, lowering blood pressure, boosting levels of HDL ('good' cholesterol), and enhancing insulin sensitivity."

Moreover, omega-3s help keep blood platelets from clinging to one another, which can defend against blood clots that may trigger a heart attack or stroke. "Thanks to their anti-inflammatory effects and their prevention of clot formation, omega-3 fatty acids help to radically reduce the incidence of cardiac rhythm disturbances as well as preserve the function of the blood vessels," says Dr. Felder.

Generally speaking, the fattier the fish, the more omega-3 fatty acids it contains, says Margo Denke, MD, associate professor of medicine in the Center for Human Nutrition at the University of Texas Southwestern Medical Center at Dallas. Interestingly, fish don't manufacture omega-3s. They derive these fats from ocean foods such as saltwater algae and other cold-water vegetation. "So cold-water trout, salmon, and mackerel are good sources of omega-3s, while farm-raised catfish isn't," says Dr. Denke. Other fish rich in omega-3 fatty acids include herring and bluefin tuna.

But fish has even more going for it than the heart-healthy omega-3 fatty acids it contains. Depending on the way it's prepared, fish is lower in dietary fat than red meat or even poultry. Three ounces of broiled or baked cod, for example, contains 89 calories, 47 grams of cholesterol, and less than 1 gram of fat.

High Marks for This School of Fish

Some of the earliest research into the heart-healthy benefits of fish dates back to studies of the Greenland Eskimos. Researchers found that despite the Eskimos' high-fat diet, they had a low incidence of heart disease, which was linked to their heavy consumption of fish.

The news has continued to be good since then. In 2004, Maggie B. Covington, MD, clinical assistant professor at the University of Maryland School of Medicine in Baltimore, published a comprehensive review of the cardiovascular benefits of omega-3 fatty acids in the journal *American Family Physician*. Her report provides a great window into the overwhelming benefits of this unique fat. Among her findings were the following:

Omega-3s can prevent sudden death in people with heart disease. Fifty to 60 percent of sudden deaths among people with heart disease are caused by ventricular arrhythmias (irregular heartbeats). But in a massive study of more than 11,000 people with heart disease (known as the GISSI-Prevenzione Trial), the group that received 850 milligrams of omega-3 fatty acids every day experienced a 45 percent reduction in sudden death and a 20 percent reduction in death overall.

Omega-3s might prevent heart attacks. Though the results have been mixed, one study in Dr. Covington's review showed that eating the

Best Choices for Omega-3s

Here's the omega-3 fatty acid content of common varieties of fish. The higher the better, when you're trolling for unwanted cholesterol.

High Levels of Omega-3s	Medium Levels of Omega-3s	Low Levels of Omega-3s
Atlantic herring	Bluefish	Atlantic cod
Atlantic mackerel	Channel catfish	Brook trout
Atlantic salmon	Halibut	Carp
Bluefin tuna	Red snapper	Flounder
Lake trout	Striped bass	Haddock
Pacific herring	Swordfish	Pacific cod
Pacific mackerel	Turbot	Rockfish
Pink salmon	Yellowfin tuna	Sole
Rainbow trout		Sturgeon
		Yellow perch
		Yellowtail

equivalent of one weekly serving of fatty fish (or about 5.5 grams of omega-3 fatty acids per month) led to a 50 percent reduction in heart attack risk.

Omega-3s can lower triglycerides and harmful LDL and raise HDL. A number of studies have been conducted on omega-3s and cholesterol, and after reviewing the results, most experts agree that omega-3s do not seem to alter total cholesterol levels. However, when taken at a level of 4 grams per day, they can reduce triglycerides by 25 to 30 percent and increase levels of "good" HDL cholesterol by 1 to 3 percent. Another study showed that taking 4 grams of omega-3s a day caused levels of VLDL (very low density lipoproteins) to drop by 30 to 40 percent.

Omega-3s can lower blood pressure. An analysis of 31 trials that included a total of 1,356 participants showed that omega-3s have a modest effect on lowering blood pressure. It seemed that levels around 4 grams a day had the greatest effect.

Falling for Fish—Hook, Line, and Sinker

The evidence in favor of fish is convincing enough that the American Heart Association has made specific recommendations: at least two servings of fish per week for people with no history of heart disease, and one serving of fish *per day* for those with known heart disease. Fish, of course, should be part of an overall cholesterol-lowering diet that includes plenty of fresh fruits and vegetables, grains, and low-fat dairy products as well as some meat and poultry.

The following tips can help you choose and prepare fish that pleases both your taste buds and your ticker.

• Stock up on canned tuna or salmon—it's an easy, inexpensive way to consume omega-3s. To save on calories, buy fish that's packed in water rather than oil. And avoid albacore tuna, which has higher-than-normal levels of mercury.

• If you're buying whole fresh fish, look for clean, tight scales; bright, clear eyes (rather than cloudy or sunken); and red or pink gills. The flesh should also spring back into place when touched.

Further, "fish should have a clean smell, not a strong odor, and the surface of the fish should be moist but not slimy," says A. Garth Rand, PhD, professor of food science at the University of Rhode Island in Kingston. Or opt for cleaned, gutted fish—it is more convenient and keeps longer, he adds.

• Unlike red meat, fish has little in the way of visible fat, so in that respect, it doesn't need trimming. But if you're preparing a fatty fish such as mackerel, tuna, or swordfish, cut away the darker flesh, says Dr. Rand. It's usually higher in fat.

• The healthiest ways to prepare fish include broiling, baking, grilling, and steaming. Don't overcook fish, however. "If the fish's moisture runs out during lengthy cooking, so will some of its nutrients," says Dr. Rand.

You might also stir-fry fish with vegetables, herbs, spices, and a small amount of low-sodium soy sauce. "Some kinds of fish make for better stir-fries than others," says Evelyn Tribole, RD, a dietitian in Beverly Hills, California, and author of *Healthy Homestyle Cooking*. "Stir-fried shrimp, lobster, and scallops are wonderful choices."

• If you love fried fish, try this healthy alternative from the American Heart Association: Dip fish fillets in flour and sauté them in a small amount of a polyunsaturated oil. Then place the fish on a heated platter, add some

---

Best Bets on Seafood Menus

Craving steamed lobster, broiled scallops, or grilled scrod? Go ahead, indulge! According to a national survey, most seafood dishes at mid-priced seafood restaurants are low in fat. It's simply a matter of angling for the right entrées.

The Center for Science in the Public Interest bought take-out portions of a variety of appetizers, side dishes, and entrées from 32 seafood restaurants across the country. The center then made a "composite" of each dish (equal portions of nine restaurants' fried fish, for example) and sent it to independent laboratories for nutritional analysis. Among the study's best-bet dishes:

- Clam chowder (1½ cups, 7 grams of fat)

- Broiled or grilled scallops (6 ounces, 3 grams of fat)

- Broiled low-fat fish such as haddock, cod, scrod, sole, or flounder (6 ounces, 5 grams of fat)

- Blackened catfish (6 ounces, 15 grams of fat)

The worst fish dishes: anything fried. That includes fish sandwiches at fast-food restaurants, say experts. "Some people believe that if they order fish sandwiches, they're taking good care of themselves," says Wahida Karmally, RD, director of nutrition at the Irving Center for Clinical Research at Columbia-Presbyterian Medical Center in New York City and a member of the American Heart Association's nutrition committee. "But eating a fish sandwich may be even worse than eating a plain burger because of all of the fat in the batter."

crushed raw garlic and lemon juice to the oil, and drizzle the seasoned oil over the fish before serving.

Or "oven-fry" fish, suggests Tribole. "Coat the fish in egg whites—no yolks—and bread crumbs, then bake until crispy," she says. "Squeeze some lemon or orange juice over the fish and sprinkle on some dill."

You might also top the fish with fresh or dried parsley, basil, tarragon, or thyme, says Tribole.

• Skewer chunks of fish, onions, tomatoes, and peppers and grill fish kebabs. "Preparing kebabs is easy, and most people enjoy them," says Tribole.

• For a quick and healthy meal, microwave fish fillets in a microwave-safe dish along with onions, mushrooms, and peppers, suggests James W. Anderson, MD, professor of medicine and clinical nutrition at the University of Kentucky College of Medicine in Lexington and author of *Dr. Anderson's High-Fiber Fitness Plan*. Or create a quick and tasty entrée by combining fish with your favorite vegetables and grains, he adds.

• If you're dining out, order a seafood appetizer. It will stoke you with omega-3s while it dampens your craving for higher-fat courses. Try boiled shrimp spritzed with lemon juice, smoked salmon served with a platter of raw vegetables, or pickled herring. (For more tips on how to order a heart-smart seafood dinner, see "Best Bets on Seafood Menus" on page 73.)

Fish Oil Supplements
A Little Extra Might Help

Many cardiovascular experts turn a skeptical eye toward nutritional supplements when it comes to reducing the risk of heart disease. While diet, exercise, and some medications have been scientifically proven to be helpful, the typical line of thinking is that most of these supplements suffer from a lack of high-quality studies.

One supplement in particular, however, has some heart experts changing their tune. The supplement is fish oil. And while the omega-3 fatty acids in fish oil (eicosapentaenoic acid, or EPA, and docosahexaenoic acid, or DHA) are common in foods, evidence has indicated that getting even more from a fish oil supplement might prove even more beneficial.

"One of the few supplements that I recommend is fish oil," says Howard N. Hodis, MD, director of the atherosclerosis research unit at the University of Southern California School of Medicine in Los Angeles. "It appears to help reduce the chances of a second heart attack, and it reduces inflammation and atherosclerosis in the arteries as well."

Why does fish oil seem to shine where other supplements have suffered? For one, people typically don't eat as much fish as is recommended, and they eat far less fish than less-healthy meats such as beef, chicken, and pork. In addition, a number of studies have shown that people can derive additional benefits by consuming levels of omega-3s that are realistic only through supplementation.

A few large studies have shown that taking around 1 gram daily of a fish oil supplement prevents death in individuals who have already experienced a heart attack. Researchers theorize that the way fish oil helps here is by preventing the arrhythmias, or irregular heartbeats, that often accompany a heart attack.

What's more, higher doses of fish oil have been shown to regulate triglyceride levels and even improve the ratio of "good" HDL cholesterol to "bad" LDL cholesterol in the bloodstream, says Christopher Speed, the director of Food and Nutrition Sciences at Ogilvy Public Relations Worldwide. "A daily dose of 4 grams of EPA plus DHA reduces triglyceride levels in the bloodstream by 25 to 30 percent," he says. "The treatment of high triglycerides always requires high doses of fish oil, around 3 to 5 grams."

When it comes to the ratio of good cholesterol to bad, fish oil seems to help primarily by boosting levels of HDL. One 8-week-long trial of 14 patients showed that supplementing approximately 2 grams of EPA and 1.5 grams of DHA led to a 40 percent increase in HDL cholesterol in the bloodstream.

Supplement Specifics

The total omega-3 fatty acid content of most fish oil supplements is around 30 percent, made up of a blend of EPA and DHA. This means you'll need to take around 3 grams of fish oil capsules to obtain 1 gram of omega-3 fatty acids.

Fish oil capsules should be taken in divided doses with meals. Though they are generally considered safe, it's always a good idea to check with your doctor before beginning any supplement regimen, particularly if you currently take a blood-thinning medication such as aspirin, heparin, warfarin, or clopidogrel. In addition, because of the risks of mercury and other environmental toxins in fish, make sure you purchase a fish oil supplement that is purified and contains an undetectable level of toxins.

Flavonoids
Food's Inner Magic

A few years ago, researchers discovered an interesting paradox when it comes to antioxidants. Nutrients that at first showed great promise for treating a number of conditions—most notably vitamins C, E, and beta-carotene—failed to live up to their medical promise when isolated in supplement form. Moreover, recent studies have shown that supplements of vitamins E and A and beta-carotene (a form of vitamin A) may do more harm than good, and even cause an increased risk of mortality.

However, the news isn't all bad when it comes to antioxidants. Rather than ruling out these nutrients completely, what researchers have learned is that the interactions between antioxidant compounds in foods are more complicated than we originally believed. It's not just the individual compounds that have heart-healthy properties, but the combinations of compounds in foods that provide maximum benefit. In fruits, vegetables, some beverages, and several other foods, antioxidant compounds known as flavonoids are part of this heart-healthy puzzle.

To date, over 4,000 flavonoids have been identified, and that may just be the tip of the proverbial iceberg. Though these compounds differ quite a bit in their molecular makeup and properties, several of them seem to exhibit a number of heart-healthy attributes when consumed in foods. "Flavonoids are a large class of phytochemicals that generally have potent antioxidant power. Many also have potent anti-inflammatory power," says Ann G. Kulze, MD, founder and CEO of Just Wellness, a wellness consulting firm in Mt. Pleasant, South Carolina, and the author of *Dr. Ann's 10-Step Diet*. "LDL cholesterol does not pose a threat to our artery walls until it is oxidized, so this combination of antioxidant and anti-inflammatory properties in flavonoids provides a great one-two punch."

A Flurry of Research

Though the research on the healthy benefits of flavonoids has been quite promising, keeping it all straight can be a bit overwhelming. Literally thousands of the compounds have been discovered in foods, and they are further classified as flavonols, flavones, flavanones, isoflavones, catechins, anthocyanidins, and chalcones based on their molecular makeup. Though vitamins C and E, selenium, and the carotenoids are the recognized dietary antioxidants, numerous recent studies have indicated that flavonoids in foods can also act as antioxidants in the body. Here is just a sampling of the recent findings on flavonoids.

One bit of news that has gotten plenty of attention of late is the heart-protective properties of red wine. Though this story doesn't appear to be about flavonoids at first glance, dig a little deeper, and you'll find that flavonoids are the story behind the story.

Sure, red wine gets some of its heart-protective properties from alcohol, which has been shown to help the heart in small amounts. But recent findings suggest something else in red wine is protecting the heart. It might just be the flavonoid compounds found in the grape seeds and grape skins that are providing the anti-clotting and antioxidant benefits. The one receiving the most buzz is a fungus-fighting chemical in the grape skins known as resveratrol. But there may be other flavonoids in red wine and grapes that are even more helpful, says John D. Folts, PhD, director of the University of Wisconsin Coronary Artery Thrombosis Research and Prevention Lab at the University of Wisconsin Hospital and Clinics in Madison. "Since there are over a thousand different kinds of flavonoids, it's going to be a major task to determine which of the flavonoids are the most significant," he says.

Another fruit that has recently shown grapelike potential is the blueberry. In 2004, researchers found a flavonoid compound in blueberries, identified as pterostilbene, that appears to lower cholesterol as effectively as the commercial drug ciprofibrate, which is sold under the name Lipanor. Though more research is needed in this area, and the exact effective dosage of pterostilbene is unknown, it certainly provides some added incentive to eat more blueberries.

Citrus fruit, particularly grapefruit, has also been making waves on the flavonoid front lately. "The primary flavonoid in grapefruit is naringin," says Gail Rampersaud, MS, RD, professor of food science and human nutrition at the University of Florida in Gainesville. "There is some experimental and epidemiological evidence that grapefruit and grapefruit juice have a positive effect on serum lipids and cardiovascular diseases."

Promising research has been popping up about the flavonoid potential of a number of other foods as well. One interesting subject is dark chocolate. Once considered a surefire diet buster, chocolate has received a new lease on life as a health food, thanks to its abundant flavonoid content. In fact, chocolate has more flavonoids than any other food! Even so, chocolate is extremely calorie dense, so you should stick to eating no more than 3 ounces of a dark chocolate bar with 60 percent cocoa or higher, says David L. Katz, MD, MPH, director of the Yale-Griffin Prevention Research Center in Derby, Connecticut, and author of *Dr. David Katz's Flavor-Full Diet*.

Tea is another food that has received a big boost, thanks to flavonoid research. Though all teas are rich in flavonoids, some research suggests that green and white teas may have more heart-healthy properties than black tea because they retain more flavonoids when being prepared. And a number of different studies have shown that regularly drinking tea appears to reduce the chances of heart disease as well as other cardiovascular risk factors.

Additional Benefits from Supplements?

Not surprisingly, all this positive news about flavonoids has inspired a wave of flavonoid supplements to hit the shelves of health food stores as well as the pages of the Internet. Can you get additional heart protection by taking a flavonoid supplement? Our experts say no. "At this time, we don't know enough about the quantities of flavonoids needed in the diet to confer optimal health benefits," says Paul F. Cancalon, PhD, of the Florida Department of Citrus in Lake Alfred, Florida. "Therefore, people should obtain flavonoids naturally from food and not through supplements since there are some indications that excessive doses may have negative effects. More research is needed to determine how flavonoids are metabolized and distributed through the body."

Get Your Fix of Flavonoids

As you can see, quite a bit of research has been conducted recently on the heart-healthy benefits of flavonoids. And, frankly, this small sampling barely scratches the surface. Scientists are discovering new foods, new flavonoids, and new benefits of these powerful antioxidant compounds all the time.

To get some sort of gauge on this flavonoid overflow, in 2006 researchers at the University of Oslo in Norway attempted to measure the antioxidant content of more than 1,000 common foods. Their findings included many of the "media darlings" that have garnered attention in recent years, such as red wine, grape juice, tea, berries, and dark chocolate, as well as a few surprising sources, such as cloves, walnuts, artichokes, pecans, cinnamon, and pineapple juice.

That's a lot of flavonoid-rich foods to keep tabs on. And trying to keep track of every flavonoid-rich food, which flavonoids it contains, and what the health benefits of those flavonoids are is a lofty pursuit even for a scientific researcher, let alone someone who is just trying to eat a heart-healthy diet.

Thankfully, making sure your diet is full of flavonoids is easier than getting a PhD in nutrition. "Eating lots of fruits and vegetables, particularly berries, and drinking wine and tea will ensure a diet high in flavonoids," says Ralph Felder, MD, PhD, section chief for cardiovascular nutrition at the Good Samaritan Medical Center in Phoenix and author of *The Bonus Years Diet*.

You may have noticed that a lot of health advisory agencies that used to say, "Eat more fruits and vegetables," now say, "Eat more *deeply colored* or *highly colored* fruits and vegetables." The reason for this is simple. As a general rule, the brighter the color, the more flavonoids a food contains. "That's why some of the best food sources include broccoli, carrots, pomegranates, citrus fruit, dark chocolate, red wine, apples, tomatoes, onions, berries, and parsley," says Dr. Kulze.

Flaxseed

A Fish Alternative?

It's fitting that "Flaxseed" falls shortly after "Fish" in the pages of this book. That's because research has shown that flaxseed may have an effect on your heart health similar to that of our water-dwelling friends. In fact, among plants, it's one of the richest sources of omega-3 fatty acids. But while the omega-3s in fish come from eicosapentaenoic acid (EPA) and docosahexaenoic acid (DHA), in flaxseed they come from linolenic acid.

In addition, flaxseed is brimming with soluble fiber, a substance also found in fresh fruits and vegetables that is known to wallop "bad" LDL cholesterol. Together, the fiber–linolenic acid offensive may clip double-digit points off your LDL cholesterol.

The Findings on Flaxseed

A number of studies have examined the effects of flaxseed on cholesterol levels, some dating back to 1993.

In the first study, conducted by the Kenneth L. Jordan Heart Foundation and Research Center in Montclair, New Jersey, 15 men and women with blood cholesterol above 240 milligrams/deciliter (mg/dl) ate three slices of bread made with flaxseed (10 percent of each loaf by weight) per day. The participants also consumed an additional 15 grams of ground flaxseed a day. After 3 months, these folks' total cholesterol took a tumble from an average of 266 to 248 mg/dl. And their LDL cholesterol fell from an average of 190 to 171 mg/dl, a 10 percent decline.

In a second study conducted by the same researchers, 13 people with moderately elevated blood cholesterol ate six slices of either wheat bread or flaxseed bread per day. In this study, flaxseed made up 30 percent of the weight of each loaf. After 6 weeks of eating the flaxseed bread, the participants' average total cholesterol fell about 10 percent, from 223 to 201 mg/dl. What's more, LDL cholesterol fell 18 percent, from 162 to 133 mg/dl—which translates into a probable reduction in heart attack risk of 30 to 40 percent. By contrast, when eating the wheat bread, the participants' total and LDL cholesterol decreased about 6 percent.

Since these early studies, a flurry of additional research has been conducted to analyze the connection between flaxseed and heart health. Most recently, researchers at the University of Manitoba in Winnipeg, Canada, looked at the effect of flaxseed on rabbits that were also fed a high-cholesterol diet. When comparing a group of rabbits that ate just the high-cholesterol diet to a group that ate the high-cholesterol diet plus flaxseed, the group of rabbits that ate the flaxseed showed significantly less damage to their arteries after

Flaxseed Bread

Makes 1 loaf; 12 slices

1½ teaspoons active dry yeast
2 tablespoons + 1¼ cups warm water
3 tablespoons honey
1 tablespoon canola oil
½ teaspoon salt
1 cup flaxseed meal
1¼ cups whole wheat flour
1¾ cups bread flour

In a large bowl, dissolve the yeast in 2 tablespoons of the water. Set aside for about 5 minutes, or until bubbly.

Mix in the honey, oil, salt, and remaining 1¼ cups water. Add the flaxseed meal, whole wheat flour, and 1 cup of the bread flour. Mix well.

Stir in enough of the remaining ¾ cup bread flour to make a soft dough. Turn out the dough onto a lightly floured surface. Knead for 10 minutes, or until smooth and elastic.

Coat a 9" x 5" loaf pan with cooking spray. Shape the dough into a loaf and place in the pan. Cover and let rise in a warm place until doubled in bulk, about 1 hour.

Bake at 350°F for 40 to 45 minutes, or until the loaf is browned on top and sounds hollow when tapped. Remove from the oven and let cool.

Per slice: 179 calories, 4.2 g total fat, 0.4 g saturated fat, 4.2 g protein, 29 g carbohydrates, 0 mg cholesterol, 3.0 g dietary fiber, 95 mg sodium

6 and 8 weeks. In addition, combining flaxseed with the high-cholesterol diet seemed to improve the relaxation response of the arteries.

Though the effects of flaxseed on cholesterol in studies have generally been positive, interestingly enough, the results with flaxseed oil supplements have been mixed. The most recent study at Emory University in Atlanta looked at 56 people who took 3 grams of flaxseed oil capsules a day. The study showed no positive benefits of taking the oil for total cholesterol, LDL, "good" HDL, or triglycerides after 26 weeks. More research is needed to determine why the results for flaxseed oil differ from flaxseed itself.

Bake a Heart-Healthy Loaf

Want to consume flaxseed as part of a low-fat, low-cholesterol diet? Bake a loaf of flaxseed bread, using the recipe on page 81.

You can buy flaxseed in many health food stores that sell grains. Grind the seeds to the consistency of cornmeal using a blender or coffee mill. As a general rule, ⅔ cup of flaxseed yields 1 cup of meal.

Flaxseed bread has a mild, nutlike taste. While it might go without saying, don't slather flaxseed bread with butter: It's too high in saturated fat. Instead, use a little jelly, or simply toast the bread and eat it plain.

Adding flaxseed to your diet may make you feel bloated and gassy, especially at first. To minimize these side effects, eat one slice of flaxseed bread a day and build up to three to six slices a day.

Fruit
Nine a Day Keep the Doctor Away

There's a simple reason that the government's most recent dietary guidelines upped the fruit and vegetable recommendation from five a day to a whopping nine: Few foods play a bigger role in our health and well-being than this dynamic duo.

Name a major health condition, and chances are fruit plays at least some role in fighting it. Cataracts, macular degeneration, cancer, high blood pressure, heart disease, and, of course, high cholesterol can all be conquered by including plentiful fruits and vegetables as part of your diet.

Fruit fights heart disease on multiple fronts. First, with only a few exceptions, it's fat free. This means it won't put anything in the bloodstream that doesn't belong there.

Fruit is also a rich source of fiber, both the insoluble and soluble kind. Insoluble fiber helps clean you out, reducing the risk of colon cancer, and soluble fiber is a heart-health superstar, as it helps carry cholesterol out of the bloodstream. The soluble fiber in most fruit is known as pectin, and it's found in abundance in grapefruit, apples, strawberries, pears, prunes, and bananas.

Of course, fruit has an incredible antioxidant potential, which also plays a role in our heart health. The most recent research seems to indicate that these antioxidants are more beneficial when derived from food rather than supplements, which is another bonus of eating whole, fresh fruit.

"In the past, the vitamin antioxidants C and E were touted frequently for their cardiovascular benefits, but clinical trials have not supported their efficacy in supplemental form," says Ann G. Kulze, MD, founder and CEO of Just Wellness, a wellness consulting firm in Mt. Pleasant, South Carolina, and the author of *Dr. Ann's 10-Step Diet*. "It now appears that food-based antioxidants are most effective. This makes perfect sense with our ever-increasing knowledge of the tens of thousands of bioactive plant compounds that appear to work together in a synergistic fashion to provide a broad range of specific disease-busting benefits, including potent antioxidant power."

That's the good news about eating more fruit. The bad news is that most people just aren't getting enough. If you don't count potatoes (which you shouldn't, as they're technically a starch), then most Americans consume only three servings of fruits and vegetables a day.

Luckily, it's easier than you think to add those extra six. To learn how—and why you want to in the first place—see the following pages.

How Fruit Fights Heart Disease

The power of fruit to keep arteries clean and stave off heart disease is backed by the weight of some of the largest medical studies in recent history. In the landmark Harvard Nurses' Health Study and Health Professionals Follow-up

Study, 110,000 men and women had their health and dietary habits recorded for 14 years. After all the results were in, the relationship between a higher intake of fruits and vegetables and a lower risk of heart disease was pretty clear. In fact, eating eight or more servings of fruits and vegetable every day corresponded with a 30 percent reduction in the risk of heart attack or stroke.

When it comes to cholesterol levels, the same amount of strong evidence exists. In the National Heart, Lung, and Blood Institute's Family Heart Study, the dietary habits of 4,466 men and women were recorded. Here again, those who ate the most fruits (four or more servings a day) had significantly lower levels of "bad" LDL cholesterol than those who ate the least. Experts are still unclear just how fruits and vegetables keep cholesterol levels down, but it could be that eating more fruit leads to eating less artery-clogging foods. Or fruits and vegetables may even play a role in blocking the absorption of cholesterol from food.

Seven Scrumptious Ways to Feast on Fruit

Sure, you can munch more apples. But there are other ways to meet your fruit quota, too. Try these juicy suggestions.

• Sample the more exotic fruits that you see at the corner fruit stand or in the produce section of your supermarket. Discovering the delights of kiwifruit, passion fruit, mangoes, pomegranates, and fresh pineapple can make eating more fruit an adventure rather than a chore.

• If you're more the classic type, treat yourself to a classic dish: fruit salad. "Slice up some melon, apples, bananas, and peaches, and top the fruits with a bit of shredded coconut," suggests Michael Klaper, MD, health director of the Royal Atlantic Health Spa in Pompano Beach, Florida, and author of *Vegan Nutrition: Pure and Simple*. (Don't overdo the coconut, though—it's very high in saturated fat.) Splash fruit juice over the salad to further boost the flavor, he says.

• Stir sliced fresh strawberries or bananas into a cup of low-fat or fat-free vanilla yogurt.

• Top pancakes or waffles (prepared with a low-fat mix) with fresh fruit, suggests James W. Anderson, MD, professor of medicine and clinical nutrition at the University of Kentucky College of Medicine in Lexington and author of *Dr. Anderson's High-Fiber Fitness Plan.* Try bananas, strawberries, fresh or frozen peaches, blueberries, or even apples sautéed with a pinch of cinnamon and nutmeg. "You can add fruit to pancake and muffin recipes, too," he says.

• Make a fruit salsa to accompany grilled chicken, fish, or turkey. Here's a simple recipe: Peel and dice half of a ripe pineapple, three kiwifruit, and half of a melon. Combine with generous amounts of chopped mint and cilantro. Let stand for at least 30 minutes before serving.

• Substitute pureed prunes for butter or margarine in homemade brownies and other chocolate baked goods, suggests Evelyn Tribole, RD, a Beverly

Heart-Healthy Indulgences

Jell-O with Fruit: Comfort Food for Cholesterol

As a child, you probably ate a gelatin dessert when you were feeling sick or just wanted a fun-to-eat treat, especially when Mom added sliced bananas or strawberries.

The best-known brand—Jell-O—has been around since 1897. If you haven't eaten gelatin for years or only make it for your kids, dig out that Jell-O mold. Paired with fruit, gelatin may help control your weight and lower your cholesterol.

Gelatin is a highly purified protein that comes from animal bones and skin. It contains no fat, carbohydrates, or cholesterol. And it's low in calories: only 80 per ½-cup serving. That's good for your heart and your weight. What's more, if you pair your favorite brand of gelatin with diced apples or various citrus fruits, the pectin in the fruits will help lower cholesterol.

Additionally, studies suggest that gelatin may help people with mild arthritic joint problems. The cartilage in joints, which is damaged by the wear and tear of arthritis, is largely made up of collagen. While trimming fat and collagenous tissue from lean meats and poultry is a healthy practice, it also means that we don't get as much collagen from foods as we used to. Adding gelatin, which is derived from collagen, to your diet may help make up for the shortfall.

Hills, California, dietitian, in her cookbook *Healthy Homestyle Cooking.* "They add a naturally sweet flavor and chewy texture," she writes. "Best yet, ½ cup of prune puree will save you nearly 800 calories and over 100 grams of fat."

• Whip up a smoothie. "Just blend your favorite fruit—say, bananas or strawberries—with some very cold water," says Dr. Klaper. These frosty blender drinks are especially refreshing on a summer day.

Fiber Up without Fattening Up

While fruit is a delicious part of a low-fat, low-cholesterol diet, you should keep the following points in mind.

First, whole fruits pack significantly more cholesterol-lowering pectin than fruit juices, says Martin Yadrick, RD, a dietitian in Manhattan Beach, California, and a spokesperson for the American Dietetic Association.

Even a pulp-filled juice can't deliver the fiber of the fruit itself, notes Yadrick. That doesn't mean you shouldn't enjoy your favorite juice; it just means that you should consume whole fruits as well.

Also, don't gorge on avocados. While this fruit is rich in monounsaturated fat, the kind that can help lower LDL cholesterol, you don't want to consume too much of any type of fat.

Happily, you can splurge on an occasional avocado, says Marilyn Cerino, RD, nutrition consultant at the Benjamin Franklin Center for Health of Pennsylvania Hospital in Philadelphia. "Many people feel that there's no substitute for really good guacamole," says Cerino. So if a rich, nutty-tasting avocado or spicy guacamole is your weakness, she says, "don't feel like you're cheating—eat it slowly and enjoy it every once in a while."

See also Antioxidants, Apples, Avocados, Berries, Fiber, Flavonoids, Oranges, Pectin, Pomegranates

Garlic

Wards Off More Than Just Vampires

Garlic is perhaps best known as a staple in Italian pasta, sauces, and other cuisine. But it's actually a popular ingredient in food all over the world. Americans consume more than 250 million pounds of this relative of the onion each year, and it's popular in Far East cuisine as well.

When you think about garlic, it usually brings to mind two things—bad breath and vampires. But research indicates that the pungent bulb may fend off more than just vampires—it may have the same effect on heart attacks and strokes.

Studies have shown that garlic appears to affect blood clots in a couple of ways. It not only seems to play a role in preventing clots from forming, it also may contribute to dissolving the clots that do form, both of which may help prevent heart attacks and strokes.

Garlic and Cholesterol

As far as cholesterol goes, garlic has been the subject of more studies than almost any other food. And the results of these studies have been mixed.

To get to the bottom of the garlic/cholesterol controversy, in 2007 the Agency for Healthcare Research and Quality (AHRQ) performed a comprehensive review of 36 different randomized trials that tested the effect of garlic on blood cholesterol levels. Their conclusion wasn't exactly a glowing recommendation of garlic. The researchers discovered that garlic appeared to have a moderate cholesterol-lowering effect when participants took it for 1 to 3 months. They concluded, however, that it was unclear whether or not the cholesterol-lowering effects could be sustained after 3 months.

The news on garlic wasn't all bad. The AHRQ researchers agreed with the assessment that garlic may play a role in reducing blood clotting and felt that more research was needed in this area.

Is this the end of the road for garlic as a cholesterol fighter? Not necessarily. But the AHRQ does recommend that consumers should be wary of garlic powder supplements that make cholesterol-lowering claims.

When it comes to food, however, there's no reason to stop adding great-tasting garlic to your favorite meals. The evidence still indicates that it might help prevent heart attacks and strokes, and it may even help cholesterol levels somewhat, as a number of studies have shown. Considering that the most common side effect of eating more garlic is just bad breath, it might be worth adding a clove or two to your favorite meals. This is one food that's worth buying extra gum or breath mints for.

Tips for Garlic Lovers

Whether you're a card-carrying garlic fan or looking for convenient ways to work this healthful seasoning into your diet, you're sure to benefit from one or more of these tips.

• "One of the easiest ways to use garlic is to chop it up, crush it, and sauté it in a little olive or canola oil," says Herbert Pierson, PhD, vice president of Preventive Nutrition Consultants in Woodinville, Wisconsin, and former project director of the Cancer Preventive Designer Food Project at the National Cancer Institute in Rockville, Maryland. "Then you can add it to soups, stews, and many other dishes that would benefit from the flavor of garlic."

• Add ground fresh garlic to salad dressings and marinades, suggests Mary Donkersloot, RD, a dietitian in Beverly Hills, California, a spokesperson for the California Dietetic Association, and author of *The Fast Food Diet*.

Getting Garlic into Your Diet—Gracefully

Try these handy strategies the next time you eat or cook with garlic.

To banish garlic breath: Love fresh garlic but hate garlic breath? Try roasting the bulbs, says Audrey Cross, PhD, associate clinical professor at Columbia University's Institute of Human Nutrition in New York City. "Roasting garlic helps reduce its odor and some of its sharpness," she says. "Brush the garlic with olive oil to keep it from drying out, then oven-roast the whole clove."

To avoid garlic-scented hands: If you want to use fresh garlic rather than the commercially prepared kind but don't want the smell clinging to your hands, consider investing in an electric chopper, suggests Janet Lepke-Harris, RD, a dietitian in Charlotte, North Carolina, and a spokesperson for the American Dietetic Association. "The garlic is chopped and ready to use in seconds," she says.

• If you'd rather not handle fresh garlic, opt for commercially prepared garlic paste or minced garlic in oil. You might also try garlic powder (made from dehydrated and pulverized cloves), garlic oil (distilled from cloves), or aged garlic extract (a water-based garlic product). One large garlic clove is equal to ½ teaspoon of garlic powder and 1 teaspoon of minced garlic. Store commercially prepared minced garlic in oil in the refrigerator and garlic powder in a cool, dark cabinet.

• Add garlic to your orange juice. Yes, you read right. "Add an odor-modified substance, such as aged garlic extract, to orange juice," says Dr. Pierson. "The juice tends to cover up even the slightest garlicky odor." His recipe: Blend three 8-ounce glasses of orange juice, a whole orange, and a tablespoon of aged garlic extract liquid.

• Don't use garlic salt. This product can be loaded with sodium, which is associated with a rise in blood pressure. What's more, garlic salt doesn't possess the health benefits of fresh garlic.

Consumed in large amounts, garlic can cause a variety of side effects, including heartburn, gas, skin irritation, and, rarely, allergic reactions in sensitive people. If you experience garlic-induced discomfort, reduce the amount of garlic you're consuming, advises Dr. Pierson. Or try cooking fresh garlic instead of eating it raw. Cooking garlic tends to weaken its irritating properties, he says.

Also, since garlic has been shown to delay blood-clotting time, consult your doctor before consuming garlic or garlic supplements if you're taking blood-thinning drugs, advises Dr. Pierson.

Grape Juice
The Breakfast Drink
of Heart Champions

By now, you have no doubt heard that red wine is good for your heart. For whatever reason, the health press has latched on to this little tidbit of news and trumpeted it from the mountaintops.

Lost in the hoopla over red wine, however, is the good news that red wine's nonalcoholic cousin, grape juice, can provide virtually the same heart-healthy benefits. And for people who don't drink, that's great news.

Just like red wine, grape juice has the ability to raise levels of "good" HDL cholesterol, while at the same time lowering the overall risk of heart disease. Grape juice also seems to prevent red blood cells from forming clots that can lead to a heart attack. Here's what the research has shown about grape juice.

The Power of Flavonoids

There's evidence to suggest that the antioxidant compounds known as flavonoids reduce the "stickiness" of blood-clotting cells, or platelets, which lowers the risk of coronary heart disease and heart attack, says John D. Folts, PhD, director of the University of Wisconsin Coronary Artery Thrombosis Research and Prevention Lab at the University of Wisconsin Hospital and Clinics in Madison. Flavonoids are found in the skin and seeds of grapes, he adds.

In research conducted at the University of Wisconsin, study participants—that is, Dr. Folts and several colleagues—drank varying amounts of grape juice. They then tested one another's blood to monitor its clotting activity. The researchers' conclusions: Purple grape juice has the same anti–clotting properties of red wine. (Dr. Folts and his colleagues used purple grape juice rather than the red or white variety because, as he says, darker juice contains more flavonoids.)

How Much Juice?

It appears to take two times as much grape juice by volume to reap red wine's preventive effects, according to Dr. Folts. "Our studies have determined that there's a measurable antiplatelet inhibition from two glasses of red wine," he says. "It takes about four glasses of grape juice to achieve the same effect." To get the most benefit from grape juice, choose dark Concord grape juice, which contains the most flavonoids and antioxidant potential.

Unfortunately, as with most heart-health remedies, grape juice isn't foolproof. "Purple grape juice has a lot of natural sugar in it, and the problem of obesity is becoming an epidemic in this country," says Dr. Folts. For that reason, it's best not to go overboard with your grape juice consumption. But a glass or two a day should be fine.

To get around the sugar issue, Dr. Folts and other researchers recently have been looking at what specific components of grapes seem to help the heart the most. Their research has narrowed it down to the grape seeds and skins. "The flavonoids in grape seeds are better antioxidants than vitamin E," says Dr. Folts. "These flavonoids may reduce heart disease risk by preventing the oxidation of 'bad' LDL cholesterol." Oxidation is a chemical process that makes LDL cholesterol more harmful and more likely to enter the arterial walls and accelerate hardening of the arteries, coronary thrombosis, and stroke.

So while grape juice can provide you with some benefit now, the purified grape seeds and skins might provide even greater benefit in the near future. "A mixture of grape seed and grape skin in capsule form is currently being studied in human subjects," says Dr. Folts. For more information on this exciting research, see page 92.

See also Alcohol, Flavonoids, Grape Seed Extract, Red Wine

Grape Seed Extract
The Cream of the Flavonoid Crop

Flavonoids, the antioxidant compounds found in some deeply colored fruits, vegetables, beverages, and other foods, may be at the cutting edge of heart-health research these days. So far, though, most studies have concluded that it's best to stick to getting flavonoids from foods, rather than trying to take flavonoid supplements.

One supplement that might just change all that, however, is grape seed extract. And when you consider how strongly the benefits of red wine, grape juice, and other grape-based products have fared under scientific testing, it should come as little surprise that a supplement with many of the same properties would perform equally well.

Grapes have been heralded for their medicinal value since the time of ancient Greece several thousand years ago. But only recently have researchers discovered that the strong healing properties of grapes and wine can be attributed directly to chemical compounds found within the grapes. One of the researchers at the forefront of studying grapes and wine over the last decade is John D. Folts, PhD, director of the University of Wisconsin Coronary Artery Thrombosis Research and Prevention Lab at the University of Wisconsin Hospital and Clinics in Madison.

In some of his earlier studies, Dr. Folts noted that both purple grape juice and red wine "reduced the 'stickiness' of blood-clotting cells, called platelets, which in turn lowered the risk of coronary heart disease and heart attack," in both animal and human studies. Through additional research, Dr. Folts discovered where exactly these heart-healthy benefits in grapes were coming from. "The flavonoids in red wine and grape juice come primarily from the seeds and skin of the grapes," he says. "These flavonoids may also reduce heart disease risk by preventing the oxidation of 'bad' LDL cholesterol."

Studies on the Seeds

In grape seed extract, supplement manufacturers have taken these flavonoids from grape seeds and packaged them in capsule form. And so far, the few studies that have been done on grape seed extract have been promising.

One study looked at the effects of grape seed extract, chromium, a combination of the two, or a placebo (an inactive pill) on blood cholesterol levels in 40 people with high cholesterol. After 2 months, the grape seed extract reduced levels of total and "bad" LDL cholesterol, but the grape seed extract combined with the chromium lowered levels even further. Another study of grape seed extract in smokers showed that the extract might prevent cholesterol from oxidizing and causing additional damage to the arteries.

The Magic of Muscadine

Though studies have yet to bear fruit, Jerry Smith, the founder and CEO of the supplement company Nature's Pearl, believes that not all grape seed extracts are created equal. His company produces a grape seed supplement made from muscadine grapes, which Smith believes contain more flavonoids and additional heart-healthy compounds than other types of grapes. So far, at least a handful of studies seem to support this claim.

"Muscadine grapes (*Vitis rotundifolia*) are genetically different from common bunch grapes (*Vitis vinifera*)," says Smith. "Muscadines have an extra pair of chromosomes (20 pairs total) that are not found in *V. vinifera* bunch grapes. Scientists believe that it is this extra genetic material that makes the muscadine so much more powerful than *V. vinifera* grapes. They can survive and thrive in the heat and humidity of the Southeast and grow wild in the woods."

According to Smith, this genetic difference also equates to a big difference in the antioxidant capacity of muscadine grapes. "There are over 100 different powerful phenolic compounds found naturally in muscadine grapes, including resveratrol, ellagic acid, quercetin, and OPCs (oligomeric proanthocyanidins), as well as a whole host of other phytochemicals that work in synergy to be antioxidant as well as anti-inflammatory," says Smith. "This is a very unique combination that isn't found in other grapes, or in other fruits or vegetables."

Of course, time will tell if Smith's muscadine grape seed supplement can live up to the hype. Nature's Pearl is currently partnering with Wake Forest University to conduct a number of human clinical trials on the effects of the supplements on various aspects of cardiovascular health, including endothelial function, inflammation, and diabetes. "These studies are being conducted as double-blind, placebo-controlled studies, which is the gold standard for clinical trials," says Smith.

So while the jury is still out on whether grape seed extract made from muscadine grapes is truly any healthier than extract made from standard grapes, stay tuned for answers. In the meantime, if you're considering trying grape seed extract as part of your cholesterol-cutting regimen, you shouldn't have too much to worry about. "The FDA has classified grape seeds as GRAS (generally regarded as safe), so they should be treated as any other foodstuff on the food pyramid," says Smith. Still, as a general rule, it's always a good idea to check with your doctor before you begin taking any dietary supplement.

Green Tea
The King of Tea . . . Or Is It?

Whether it's chamomile, peppermint, or another natural blend, herbalists have been recommending brews of herbal tea to cure what ails us for hundreds, if not thousands, of years. Recently, however, it seems that tea—or *Camellia sinensis*, for the scientists out there—may be the most powerful healer of all.

Name a health condition of concern to the general population, and chances are good you'll find a study that says tea has a hand in healing it. Research indicates that green tea might prevent cervical, breast, and prostate cancers, not to mention cancers of the liver and digestive system, and certain types of leukemia. And for cancer patients taking chemotherapy or radiation, green tea can keep their white blood cell counts up.

Green tea can also help people lose weight, protect their skin, and preserve the immune system—and we haven't even talked about the heart yet!

When it comes to the heart, green tea is no less remarkable. A number of studies seem to indicate that green tea can lower total cholesterol, "bad" LDL cholesterol, and triglycerides, not to mention raise levels of "good" HDL cholesterol. And because green tea is positively loaded with heart-healthy antioxidants, it can prevent cholesterol from oxidizing in the bloodstream and contributing to atherosclerosis. It may even play a role in diabetes treatment.

What's Up with Green?

You may have noticed by now that among this laundry list of conditions that tea can help with, the word "tea" in all instances is preceded by the word "green." In actuality, the three main types of tea—black, oolong, and green—all come from the same plant: the previously mentioned *Camellia sinensis*.

So, you might ask, if all these teas are from the same plant, wouldn't they have the same healthy properties? You'd think so, but the way these teas are processed leads to the differences. Black teas and oolong teas are fermented to some degree, which destroys a number of their active ingredients. Green tea, on the other hand, is not fermented at all. As a result, it's positively brimming with heart-healthy ingredients.

The Muscle behind Tea

These ingredients, as it turns out, are flavonoids, the same plant-based antioxidant compounds discussed in detail on page 76. In green tea, though, the flavonoids are known as polyphenols. The polyphenols are what give tea its bitter taste, but they also give it antioxidant potential that's greater than even vitamin C.

Not to bog you down in too much science here, but you may have noticed that a lot of teas these days are hyping their "EGCG" content. EGCG, or epigallocatechin gallate, is the most studied polyphenol in green tea and also the most active. Much of green tea's miraculous healing potential has been

---

White Tea—Green's Heir to the Throne?

Just when it looked like green tea might be the ultimate health food, it seems that it already may have been supplanted by its own brother (or is that sister?)—white tea.

As with black and oolong teas, the difference between white tea and green tea is the way they are processed. While green tea is allowed to mature and then air-dry before it is prepared for sale, white tea leaves and buds are picked when they are very young, and then they are immediately steamed to preserve the polyphenol content within. As a result, studies have shown that the flavonoid and polyphenol content of white tea is even higher than that of green tea.

Though it's still too early to determine if white tea is any more effective than green tea as a heart healer or cholesterol cutter, it stands to reason that white tea would have similar effects. So while the studies are still under way, feel free to break up the monotony of drinking green tea with the occasional white one. Your heart will thank you later.

attributed to EGCG, and there are even EGCG supplements on the market. More research is still needed to determine the effectiveness of these supplements, though.

The Green Scene

Break green tea down to its pure, brewed form, or a "green tea extract" form, and the evidence seems pretty compelling that it can play a role in lowering cholesterol levels. Most recently, a 2003 study had 240 men and women with mild-to-moderate high cholesterol take either 375 milligrams of green tea extract or a placebo (an inactive pill) every day. After 12 weeks, those taking the green tea extract lowered total cholesterol by 11 percent and LDL cholesterol by 16 percent, and raised HDL cholesterol by 2 percent.

Japanese researchers investigated the link between green tea intake and cardiovascular and liver diseases in 1,371 men over age 40. The researchers found that as tea consumption rose, "good" HDL cholesterol increased, while levels of triglycerides (another blood fat implicated in heart disease), total cholesterol, and LDL cholesterol fell. In fact, total cholesterol in the men who drank 10 or more cups of tea a day was about 6 percent lower than in the men who drank three or fewer cups a day.

In another Japanese study of 1,300 men, researchers found that the greater the consumption of green tea, the lower the men's cholesterol. Men who drank two or fewer cups of tea a day had total cholesterol levels averaging 193 milligrams/deciliter (mg/dl). Those who drank between six and eight cups a day had an average cholesterol reading of 188 mg/dl. And the average cholesterol of men who drank nine or more cups a day was even lower—185 mg/dl.

Tea and Supplements

Nine or more cups of green tea a day may seem a bit extreme. Luckily, most experts agree that drinking a much more realistic two to three cups of green tea a day will provide some benefit—not to mention a whopping 240 to 320 milligrams of polyphenols. Green tea extract has garnered favor among many in the medical community as well. If you'd like to try the extract, 300 to 400 milligrams per day of a standardized green tea extract is recommended. Just be sure to talk to your doctor before starting this or any supplement regimen.

Lean Meat

The Red Scare Is Over

When it comes to high cholesterol, red meat definitely takes more heat than it does from a charcoal grill. Thanks to its saturated fat content, which has been shown to raise cholesterol levels, it's often portrayed as "public enemy number one" in the war on cholesterol.

But is the criticism really justified? After all, red meat has a lot of things that are good for your body. It's a great source of protein, iron, zinc, and B vitamins. Plus, a little bit of saturated fat is necessary for the body to function properly. The phospholipids created from saturated fatty acids are actually critical to the formation of healthy cell membranes.

The problem, as with many things in the American diet, is that most people get too much. That's why the American Heart Association recommends that less than 7 percent of your daily caloric intake should come from saturated fats.

Sound tricky? It's really easier than you think, and it takes only two steps to get there. Step one is to eat smaller portions of red meat. And that means cutting out the monster 16-ounce porterhouse you might enjoy from time to time. In reality, a serving of beef should be about 3 ounces cooked—which is about the size of a deck of cards. If this doesn't sound like enough, don't worry. We have some tips to create satisfying meals with this much beef on page 99.

Step two in reducing saturated fat intake is to eat leaner cuts. And thanks to some help from the nation's beef producers, this is easier than ever before.

Take a stroll through the grocery store these days, and you'll probably notice that steaks have a lot less fat hanging from the edges than in years past. You'll also notice that you can get ground beef that's 90, 93, and even 96 percent lean.

This is no accident. When American consumption of red meat plummeted in the 1980s, the nation's beef producers stepped up their efforts to create a product that was desirable to the more health-conscious American. They crossbred cattle with leaner animals, gave them lower-fat feed, and sent them to market younger, when their beef was less fatty. Also, butchers began trimming more fat from the meat right in the supermarket or butcher shop.

The result is that beef has actually become lower in fat, cholesterol, and calories than it used to be. Moreover, "some of the leaner cuts of red meat contain less fat than skinless chicken thighs," says Tammy Baker, RD, general manager for the Dairy Council of Arizona and former spokesperson for the American Dietetic Association.

No Beef with Beef

A few studies have beefed up the argument that red meat can be part of a cholesterol-lowering diet.

In a study at Baylor College of Medicine in Houston, two groups of men with high blood cholesterol levels were placed on a 5-week stabilization diet in which 40 percent of their calories came from fat. These men then switched to one of two low-fat test diets in which they ate either chicken breast or lean beef (choice strip loin steak) for 5 more weeks. The beef contained 8 percent fat, and the chicken, 7 percent fat.

After 5 weeks, both groups' total cholesterol decreased significantly—7.6 percent for the meat eaters and 10.2 percent for the poultry eaters. The men's "bad" LDL cholesterol also dropped significantly on both diets, although not

The Kindest Cuts

The following cuts of beef are among the leanest. Figures are for 3 ounces cooked. For comparison, the same amount of rib eye steak contains 10 grams of fat and 191 calories, and 3 ounces of short ribs packs 15.4 grams of fat and 251 calories.

Meat	Fat (g)	Calories
Eye of round	4.2	143
Top roast	4.2	153
Tip round	5.9	157
Top sirloin	6.1	165
Chuck roast	7.6	189
Top loin	8	176
Flank	8.6	176
Tenderloin	8.6	177

to desirable levels. The researchers concluded that lean beef and chicken are interchangeable in a low-fat, low-cholesterol diet.

In an Australian study, researchers placed 10 people on a very low-fat diet that contained lean beef with the fat trimmed off. The participants' total cholesterol fell significantly within a week. But when beef fat (in the form of drippings) was added to these folks' diet, their total cholesterol rose. The researchers concluded that it was the beef fat, not the beef itself, that raised blood cholesterol. Further, they wrote, the low-fat diet with lean beef (but without the fat drippings) was just as effective at lowering cholesterol as other low-fat diets that were tested.

A Carnivore's Guide to Cholesterol Busting

To make red meat part of your low-fat, low-cholesterol diet, keep these shopping guidelines and serving suggestions in mind.

- Choose the leanest cuts of meat. If you're shopping for pork, select the tenderloin, leg, and shoulder. If you're buying lamb, choose the arm and loin.

- For steaks, go with the label "USDA select," and for ground beef, choose "extra lean." On average, select beef contains 20 percent less fat than "choice" beef and 40 percent less fat than "prime." "Extra-lean" ground beef contains just 10 percent fat based on weight.

- You can estimate the fat content of a cut of meat just by looking at it, according to Mary Donkersloot, RD, a dietitian in Beverly Hills, California, a spokesperson for the California Dietetic Association, and author of *The Fast Food Diet*. "Check to see how much white marbling the meat has," she suggests. The more marbling, she says, the more fat.

- Cut away all visible fat from red meat before you cook it. While trimming the fat won't affect its taste much, it will dramatically reduce your intake of fat and calories.

- "If you eat meat, broil it," suggests Gene A. Spiller, DSc, PhD, director of the Health Research and Studies Center in Los Altos, California, and author of *The Superpyramid Eating Program*. "Let the fat drip off the meat, but don't let it drain on hot charcoal or a hot burner, which will create undesirable fumes."

• If you're wondering how to make do with a 3-ounce serving of meat, get creative. Three ounces might look pretty wimpy as a steak by itself, but if you add it to a stir-fry dish, mix it into a stew with a bounty of vegetables, or top a delicious salad with it, suddenly it starts to look like a satisfying meal. Other options are to use 3 ounces of ground beef in spaghetti sauce, or make a low-fat beef stroganoff dish.

• Eat red meat in moderation. To help you with this goal, you can substitute whole or ground turkey or chicken in recipes that call for beef. Make turkey burgers instead of hamburgers, or meat loaf with ground turkey instead of ground beef.

"But the less fatty the meat, the drier it can get," says Evelyn Tribole, RD, a dietitian in Beverly Hills, California, and author of *Healthy Home-style Cooking.* She suggests adding a medium-size grated apple to a pound of ground turkey. "The apple will give the turkey a nice texture without adding extra fat," she says.

Heart-Healthy Indulgences

Chili con Carne: The Perfect Way to Enjoy Beef

Eating the right kind of beef—in moderate amounts—can help lower your cholesterol levels, according to a study conducted at three different American research institutions.

One study looked at 202 men and women with mildly to moderately elevated cholesterol levels. For 9 months, 5 to 7 days a week, half of them followed a heart-healthy diet, with lean beef making up 80 percent of the meat they ate. The others ate lean chicken breast for the same period. Both groups lowered their cholesterol—almost 8 percent for the meat eaters and a little over 10 percent for the poultry eaters. The researchers concluded that lean beef and chicken are interchangeable in a low-fat, low-cholesterol diet.

For an inexpensive, convenient, heart-healthy meal, make chili con carne. Combine lean ground beef (sautéed and drained of excess fat), fiber-rich kidney beans, and cholesterol-lowering garlic, along with tomatoes, onions, and zesty seasonings such as cumin, chili powder, and oregano.

• "Marinate meat in something flavorful," suggests Marilyn Cerino, RD, nutrition consultant at the Benjamin Franklin Center for Health of Pennsylvania Hospital in Philadelphia. A savory marinade is a blend of fresh orange juice, light soy sauce, olive oil, garlic, and ginger. "You can use this mixture to marinate strips of meat or chicken that you plan to stir-fry," says Cerino. "And if the meat is tough, marinate it overnight."

• You can make the classic American hamburger and its traditional side dishes a lot healthier meal with just a few simple changes. Choose "extra-lean" ground beef for the burger, substitute a whole grain bun for a white-bread bun, and use low-fat or cholesterol-free mayonnaise and low-fat or fat-free cheese instead of regular mayo and American cheese. Put away your deep-fat fryer and opt for spiced, oven-baked home fries (or sweet potato fries) instead. Round out the meal with a side dish of baked beans without the salt pork—lots of fiber, virtually no fat.

• If you must have a fast-food burger, order a small burger without fixings such as cheese, mayonnaise, and special sauce, suggests Baker. On the side, opt for a salad with low-fat or fat-free dressing or a baked potato without sour cream or butter.

Low-Fat and Fat-Free Cheeses

Enjoy Rich Flavor— Without All the Fat

If red meat is thought to be the "Bonnie" of heart health, then cheese just might be the "Clyde." Once considered a healthy part of anyone's diet, cheese has now been relegated to the same blacklist occupied by the meat of the animal that produces it. It sure seems hard to be a cow these days.

The reason that cheese has been blackballed? No food in our standard diet has a higher concentration of saturated fat than cheese does. And too much saturated fat has been shown to raise levels of total cholesterol and "bad" LDL cholesterol.

Unfortunately, the numbers don't lie. The latest "Dietary Guidelines for Americans," published in 2005, recommend that most people limit their saturated fat intake to under 20 grams a day. And a measly 1 ounce of regular Cheddar cheese will give you almost one-third of that, or 6 grams, right off the bat.

As you can see, it doesn't take much cheese to shoot your heart-healthy diet right out of the water. In fact, the government has estimated that cheese is the *number one* contributor of saturated fat to the modern American diet, surpassing even beef. A whopping 13.1 percent of the saturated fat we consume comes from cheese.

Luckily, the news about cheese isn't all bad. Despite the drawbacks, it's still a rich source of protein and calcium. And just as with red meat, dairies have responded to the public's concerns by offering a variety of low-fat and even fat-free cheeses that have the benefits and flavor of cheese without all the fat. One ounce of low-fat Cheddar cheese, for example, contains just 1.2 grams of fat and only 49 calories.

While you'll never mistake a low-fat cheese for your favorite Brie or Camembert, you can still enjoy rich, flavorful meals and snacks with cheese by using just a bit of creativity. We talked to a number of experts to help you select the right cheeses and prepare them in heart-healthy ways.

Smart Strategies for Choosing Cheese

The key to choosing heart-healthy cheese, say experts, is to become a dedicated label reader. Select cheeses with low amounts of total fat and saturated fat and low percentages of calories from fat, advises Sheah Rarback, RD, director of nutrition at the Mailman Center at the University of Miami School of Medicine.

"Choose a cheese in which the percentage of fat is lower than the percentage of protein," says Gene Spiller, DSc, PhD, director of the Health Research and Studies Center in Los Altos, California, and author of *The Superpyramid Eating Program*. A product that is 20 percent fat and 15 percent protein, for example, should stay out of your shopping cart, he says.

Also, don't be fooled by cheese's relatively low level of dietary cholesterol. At first glance, the 26 milligrams of cholesterol in a 1-ounce serving of American cheese barely makes a dent in the 300 milligrams of daily dietary cholesterol that the American Heart Association says is acceptable. But what's really important here is saturated fat. That same serving of cheese packs a whopping 9 grams of saturated fat, almost half of the recommended daily limit of 20 grams.

Finally, what cheese you choose really comes down to how much you consume in the first place. "If a person is a high consumer of cheese, using lower-fat cheese is essential," says Alicia Moag-Stahlberg, RD, a dietitian with Action for Healthy Kids, a nonprofit organization located in Chicago whose mission is to improve children's nutrition and physical activity. "If someone has only one to two servings of cheese a week, though, some regular cheese can be incorporated into the diet."

Low-Fat or Fat-Free?

If you're looking to knock a few points off your blood cholesterol by slicing your intake of fatty cheese, you might try low-fat or fat-free cheeses. Here's how these products compare.

Low-fat cheeses. At 3 grams or less of fat per ounce and 20 to 50 percent less fat than full-fat cheeses, these products look and taste much like their higher-fat counterparts, says Moag-Stahlberg. Low-fat products even melt like their full-fat counterparts, making them perfect for sauces and toasted

---

A Tip from the French

Just can't give up your favorite full-fat cheese? You might try doing as the French—the world's most prolific cheese eaters—do, says Audrey Cross, PhD, associate clinical professor at Columbia University's Institute of Human Nutrition in New York City.

"The French eat very high-fat cheeses," says Dr. Cross. "But they eat tiny amounts of them, along with a lot of bread and fruit. Americans tend to eat hunk after hunk of cheeses that aren't as satisfying, trying to attain some satisfaction.

"If we would eat foods that taste good, we'd eat less of them, because we'd be satisfied," continues Dr. Cross. "Try eating an ounce of your favorite cheese instead of 5 ounces of a variety that you don't enjoy as much. And eat the cheese with bread and a piece of fruit instead of with fatty crackers."

cheese sandwiches. "Most people are quite happy with low-fat cheeses," she adds. If you're already following a low-fat diet, you may want to select a low-fat cheese over a fat-free product.

Fat-free cheeses. The good news about fat-free cheeses is that they've been stripped of all but a trace amount of fat, so they're good for your heart. The bad news? That fat is what gives cheese its texture, flavor, and consistency in the first place. This means that fat-free cheese will be, shall we say, an acquired taste for people who are accustomed to full-fat cheeses. And others might just find it flat-out bland. It also doesn't melt quite as nicely as other kinds of cheese.

Heart-Healthy Indulgences

Gorgonzola and Cheddar Cheese: Strong Flavor, Big Benefits

In small amounts, cheese can be a diet good guy.

A 1½-ounce serving of Cheddar offers about 300 milligrams of calcium, as much as a glass of milk. Cheese also contains a type of fat called conjugated linoleic acid, or CLA, which scientists are investigating as a new weapon against breast cancer. Additionally, eating cheese at the end of meals can protect your teeth against decay.

Still, all this good news comes with a gentle reminder that cheese has a lot of saturated fat. That 1½-ounce serving packs 9 grams of it, and that's not great for your heart. So, while we're not telling you to cut cheese out of your heart-healthy diet altogether, it's best to consume it in small portions. Experts suggest choosing extra-sharp Cheddar or Gorgonzola because their strong flavors will satisfy your taste buds in smaller amounts.

Here are some other tips for indulging in real cheese.

Know your Gorgonzola. Be on the lookout for it at the next party you attend, or serve it at your own bash. Gorgonzola has a light ivory surface, and its interior is marbled with blue-green veins. The American Dairy Association says that it tastes great with sweet crackers and walnuts (which are well-known for their cholesterol-cutting power).

Avoid temptation. At home, help yourself to one serving of cheese, then wrap the rest and store it right away.

While fat-free cheese might not be the ideal choice for some dishes, you can create flavorful meals using fat-free cheese with just a little creativity. The secret is to pair it with other ingredients in salads, sandwiches, and other dishes, so that the various flavors can enhance that of the cheese.

Tasty Tips for Cheese Junkies

The kind of cheese you choose—and the way you use it—can make all the difference. These hints can help.

• Look for low-fat "impostors." Chances are there's a low-fat or fat-free alternative for your favorite type of full-fat cheese, including Cheddar (Healthy Choice Fat-Free, Cracker Barrel Light), mozzarella (Kraft Healthy Favorites, Alpine Lace Low Moisture Part-Skim), Swiss (Light 'n' Lively Singles, Kraft Light Naturals) and American (Weight Watchers Slices, Kraft Free Singles).

"Do some taste testing," says Evelyn Tribole, RD, a dietitian in Beverly Hills, California, and author of *Healthy Homestyle Cooking*. "You may find that there's a considerable difference in taste among brands of the same type of cheese."

• Try combining small amounts of a higher-fat cheese with a low-fat or fat-free product. "You might add cubes of low-fat mozzarella to a salad, and then sprinkle the salad with blue cheese," says Ruth Lowenberg, RD, a dietitian in New York City. "You'll get a wonderful cheesy flavor without using a large amount of the higher-fat cheese."

• Using condiments can give a fat-free cheese some extra zip. "If you're using a fat-free cheese in a sandwich, you may not be able to get away with adding just lettuce and tomato," says Lowenberg. "Try spreading on some horseradish or chutney, which will enhance the cheese's flavor."

• To make a delicious dip, blend some 2% cottage cheese with a dry salad-dressing mix, suggests Lowenberg. If a dip recipe calls for sour cream, substitute a mixture of 2% cottage cheese and low-fat yogurt, she says.

• Substitute fat-free cream cheese for the full-fat product in no-bake cheesecakes and refrigerated desserts. Or toss fat-free cream cheese with hot pasta (along with your favorite herbs and spices) for a creamy, Alfredo-type sauce.

• Love the taste of creamy cheeses such as Brie? Mix one part Brie cheese, four parts fat-free cream cheese, and some rosemary, shape into rounds, and dip in bread crumbs. Then bake.

• The next time you make lasagna, substitute reduced-fat ricotta cheese for the whole-milk product. A half-cup of reduced-fat ricotta contains 9.8 grams of fat, compared with 16.1 grams in the same amount of the whole-milk stuff.

• As mentioned previously, fat-free cheeses don't melt very well. So don't use these products to top casseroles, advises Tribole. "Fat-free cheese will look like toasted coconut," she says. "I'd use a low-fat cheese instead." Similarly, fat-free mozzarella works better baked into lasagna than on a pizza, she notes. But if you want to use a fat-free cheese in a sauce, "try shredding it very finely," Tribole suggests. "It will melt nicely."

Meal Frequency
More Meals = Better Heart Health

If someone told you that eating more meals more often could not only help you lose weight but also lower your cholesterol, you'd probably think they were pulling your leg. But then you'd probably want to know more. After all, who wouldn't want to hear great news like this?

But as crazy as it sounds, a growing number of studies have shown that it's actually true. Eating smaller meals more frequently throughout the day can leave you more satisfied—and less likely to blow your diet by gorging yourself when lunch or dinner rolls around. There's even a name for this approach to eating—grazing.

In a South African study, for example, men who ate breakfast as smaller "mini-meals" throughout the morning then ate 27 percent less at lunch than men who ate one large breakfast. And that, in turn, can lead to weight loss and a few points falling off your cholesterol level.

But before you get ready to chow down, be aware that grazing, just like eating any meals, takes some discipline. Getting the green light to eat more often shouldn't mean that you start filling in your usual diet with fatty desserts and treats. Remember, the idea here is *smaller* meals more often. It's more meals, not more calories.

At the same time, your new "meals" don't necessarily have to be carrot and celery sticks (although those wouldn't be bad choices). Studies indicate that individuals can benefit from this approach to eating, even if they're munching on the same foods as they did before.

It Pays to Graze

Grazing may be the natural way to eat, says Elizabeth Barrett-Connor, MD, professor and chairperson of the department of family medicine at the University of California, San Diego. "We evolved from people who ate frequent, small meals when they could," she says. "Occasionally, they would get a big kill and gorge. But Americans gorge nearly every night—and that's an unhealthy way to eat."

The body manages smaller meals more efficiently, explains Sharon Edelstein, a research scientist at George Washington University in Washington, D.C. "Humans were meant to be grazers, and that's the way our bodies perform best," she says. "If you pound your body with a lot of food once or twice a day, you may be giving it too much to deal with. If you put food into your body more slowly, you'll process it more efficiently."

Dr. Barrett-Connor agrees. "Eating more meals consisting of less food is more physiologically efficient," she says. "If you throw large amounts of fat and calories at the body all at once, it won't be able to manage them as well. It's more than the body can metabolize." So fueling up only once or twice a day may make it easier for dietary fat to collect in the coronary arteries, leading to elevated cholesterol levels, she says.

If you'd like more evidence that eating smaller portions may affect heart health, Marla Mendelson, MD, assistant professor of medicine at Northwestern University Feinberg School of Medicine in Chicago, suggests looking at countries that have lower incidences of cardiovascular disease than the United States, such as Japan and China. "The people in these countries eat smaller portions," says Dr. Mendelson. "This may aid the digestive process, so you're not completely overwhelming the mechanism in the liver with too much food and asking the liver to process it." Overloading the liver with food may eventually cause free-floating fat and cholesterol to be deposited in the arteries, she says.

Four (or More) Meals Are Better Than One

Scientific research seems to support the notion that smaller, more frequent meals can help out your heart. Edelstein and Dr. Barrett-Connor, along with other colleagues, studied the diets of more than 2,000 people. They found that the total cholesterol of people who ate four or more meals a day was almost 9 points lower than that of the people who reported eating one or two meals a day, says Dr. Barrett-Connor. Also, the frequent eaters' "bad" LDL cholesterol averaged 6 points lower than that of the infrequent eaters, she says. And while the grazers tended to consume more fat, calories, and cholesterol than the two-meal group, their blood cholesterol was still lower, and they were less likely to be obese.

Researchers in New Zealand had 19 healthy men and women with normal blood cholesterol levels consume their usual low-fat diets—with one difference: These folks alternated between eating three meals a day and eating nine meals a day. They spent 2 weeks on each diet. When the participants followed the nine-meal plan, their total cholesterol fell 6.5 percent, and their LDL cholesterol dropped 8.1 percent. If every 1 percent change in total cholesterol translates to a 2 percent change in the risk of coronary heart disease, wrote the researchers, "then theoretically, there could be a mean 13 percent reduction in the risk of coronary heart disease when meal frequency is increased from three to nine meals a day."

Eat Like a Bird—All Day

Thinking of joining the graze craze? These tips can help.

- Work your way up gradually. For the standard meal eater, switching to five or six meals a day can be overwhelming. So start by reducing the size of your regular meals and working in a healthy snack between meals until you get the hang of it.

- Get groceries for grazing. By planning your weekly foods and sticking to that list, you can get healthy foods for your small meals that will be properly portioned for your needs.

- Erase empty calories. The problem with most snacks is that they often consist of high-fat, high-sugar foods with no nutritional value. But if your snacks become fruits, vegetables, nuts, and other healthy choices, you'll be deriving some healthy benefits—and feel more satisfied and less likely to gorge when the next meal rolls around.

Mediterranean Diet

Rich Food—Heart-Healthy Results

If you think eating for your heart health means eating boring, bland foods, then you'll love this news. You can enjoy a diet that's even richer than a standard American diet—brimming with fresh fish and seafood, rich sauces, delicious fruits and vegetables, and hearty olive oil—and lower your risk of high cholesterol and heart disease.

Sound too good to be true? For centuries, these foods have been the staples of the diets of the French, Italians, Greeks, and Spanish as well as other people living in Mediterranean countries. And the results of that diet are hard to refute: People in these countries are much less likely to die of heart disease or heart attack than Americans. In fact, while 107 out of every 100,000 people in the United States die of heart disease, the number drops to just 69 for Greece, 65 for the Italians, 54 for the Spanish, and 40 for the French.

The evidence is strong enough that the American Heart Association decided to test the effectiveness of the Mediterranean diet in the landmark Lyon Diet Heart Study. In this study, 605 heart attack survivors were divided into two groups. One group followed a Mediterranean-style diet that featured abundant amounts of bread, root vegetables, green vegetables, fruit, and fish. It also was low in red meat, lamb, butter, and cream. The other group received no dietary advice but was told by their physicians to follow a "prudent" diet.

The results of the study were quite significant. The researchers estimated that after 46 months of following the Mediterranean diet, the Mediterranean diet group had lowered their risk of heart disease by 50 to 70 percent. Though other healthy lifestyle choices (such as activity level) and other risk factors (such as smoking) may have played a role in this outcome, the Mediterranean diet definitely had a significant impact on the results.

Secrets of the Sea

How can such a rich, hearty diet have such a positive benefit on heart health? As it turns out, when you break the Mediterranean diet down to its individual components, most of them have been shown to benefit the heart on their own. Olive oil is a healthy source of monounsaturated fat, which can maintain or even slightly increase levels of "good" HDL cholesterol. Fish are rich in omega-3 fatty acids that help the heart in a number of ways, including lowering triglyceride levels and reducing the formation of clots. And fruits, vegetables, and beans are rich in fiber and antioxidants. Put all these together in meals that are rich, flavorful, and fun to eat, and you can see why the Mediterranean diet has heart experts so excited.

As it turns out, though, the diet may be just as effective for what it *doesn't* have—namely, high levels of saturated fat from foods such as red meat, butter, cream, and cheese. In fact, the American Heart Association says that the typical Mediterranean diet has many of the same properties of the two diets that they already recommend to reduce the risk of heart disease: the Eating Plan for Healthy Americans and the TLC (Total Lifestyle Change) diets.

A Prudent—But Not Spartan—Cuisine

At first glance, the Mediterranean diet appears to be just as reliant on fat as the American one. But when you look a little closer at the type of fat consumed, the difference becomes crystal clear.

The traditional Mediterranean diet averages 35 to 40 percent of total calories from fat. So does the typical American diet. But the American diet is laden with artery-clogging saturated fat, found in animal-derived foods such as red meat, in whole-milk dairy products, and in processed convenience foods. Mediterranean cuisine, on the other hand, tends to be richer in artery-

Salut—In Moderation

In Italy, France, and Greece, a bottle of red wine is as much a part of a meal as the robust cuisine and the hearty laughter around the table. But if you don't drink, don't start for the sake of your heart, say experts.

"I advise people to limit their intake of alcohol to seven drinks a week," says James W. Anderson, MD, professor of medicine and clinical nutrition at the University of Kentucky College of Medicine in Lexington and author of *Dr. Anderson's High-Fiber Fitness Plan*. (A drink is frequently defined as 4 ounces of wine, 12 ounces of beer, or $1\frac{1}{2}$ ounces of liquor.)

Should you opt to enjoy an occasional glass of vino, there's no need to fret about the wine's year or its bouquet. When it comes to wine's apparent heart-healthy benefits, an inexpensive California Chablis is just as good as the priciest French Bordeaux.

saving monounsaturated fat, particularly olive oil. In the Mediterranean region, the per-capita consumption of olive oil has averaged as high as 2 to 3 tablespoons per day. The typical American, on the other hand, consumes about 3 tablespoons of olive oil every 4 months. But given the popularity of low-fat cooking and a cholesterol-conscious population, Americans might use more olive oil in the near future.

In an editorial in the *New England Journal of Medicine*, Walter Willett, MD, DrPH, professor of epidemiology and nutrition at the Harvard School of Public Health, and his colleague Frank M. Sacks, MD, professor of medicine and nutrition, endorsed the traditional Mediterranean diet, saying that it's just as low in saturated fat and cholesterol as a typical low-fat diet. The Mediterranean alternative—using monounsaturated fat as a major dietary component—is now shown to be more healthful than following a low-fat diet and may be an even better way to improve blood cholesterol and blood pressure levels. Further, they wrote, eating the Mediterranean way "will provide more variety and greater satisfaction to many." That's good news for those of us with higher-than-average cholesterol—and hearty appetites.

Eat as in Rome—At Home

If you're accustomed to a diet of beef and butter, the Mediterranean diet may seem a little . . . well, foreign. But many Americans have found that Mediterranean cuisine is as delicious and inexpensive as it is health promoting. Here's how to add the Mediterranean touch to your table.

- Eat less red meat. "In Italy, the focus of the meal is pasta, and meat is more of a side dish," says Wahida Karmally, RD, director of nutrition at the Irving Center for Clinical Research at Columbia-Presbyterian Medical Center in New York City and a member of the American Heart Association's nutrition committee. "By following the Italian approach and consuming less meat, you can reduce your intake of saturated fat."

- Replace butter and other saturated fats with monounsaturated fat, particularly olive oil. Drizzle this fragrant oil over pasta, steamed vegetables, and baked potatoes, for example. Or use it to sauté onions and vegetables. Better yet, use an olive oil cooking spray.

- Eat more fresh vegetables. They're packed with cholesterol-reducing soluble fiber and antioxidants, which experts speculate may help keep "bad"

LDL cholesterol from a damaging chemical reaction called oxidation. (Oxidized LDL becomes stickier and clings to artery walls, experts theorize.) Prepare a French-style ratatouille (an eggplant-based vegetable stew) by simmering onions, eggplant, zucchini, and tomatoes with herbs and spices. Serve with crusty French bread, sans butter.

• Consume more whole grains, advises James W. Anderson, MD, professor of medicine and clinical nutrition at the University of Kentucky College of Medicine in Lexington and author of *Dr. Anderson's High-Fiber Fitness Plan*. Some varieties, such as barley and oats, are packed with soluble fiber. Try whole wheat pasta rather than the white-flour variety, suggests Dr. Anderson. Or you might try combining seasoned vegetables with bulgur or couscous (which contain more fiber than white rice) to make a spicy Spanish-style pilaf.

• Eat more legumes. Chickpeas, lentils, and white beans, mainstays of Mediterranean cuisine, are great sources of low-fat protein and are rich in soluble fiber. Try the classic Italian dish *pasta e fagioli* (pasta with beans) or enjoy a French-style white-bean salad.

• Use more garlic. Besides adding its distinctive flavor and aroma to foods, this aromatic herb may contain certain components that help lower choles-

The Mediterranean Diet Pyramid

The Harvard School of Public Health, the Oldways Preservational and Exchange Trust, and the World Health Organization Regional Office for Europe have endorsed the Mediterranean Diet Pyramid. This dietary model, an alternative to the USDA Food Guide Pyramid, is modeled on the traditional diets of the Mediterranean region around 1960 (before heavy influences from other nations).

At the base of the pyramid is daily physical activity. On the next two levels are foods that are eaten daily and in abundance: breads, cereals, and grains; fruits and vegetables; and beans, other legumes, and nuts. The next two levels contain foods that are eaten daily but in low to moderate amounts: olive oil and cheese and yogurt. (Olive oil should become the principal fat in your diet, replacing other fats and oils.)

The next four levels are foods that are eaten only a few times per week and in low to moderate amounts: fish, poultry, eggs, and sweets.

At the top of the pyramid is red meat, which is consumed only a few times per month.

Further, the Mediterranean Diet Pyramid suggests drinking six glasses of water per day and consuming wine in moderate amounts each day (if at all).

terol. Add minced garlic to pasta dishes, soups and stews, sauces, and grilled fish. Or whip up a pot of garlic broth, a popular French staple. Peel and slice six cloves of garlic. Place them in a 1-quart saucepan with 2 cups of water, one bay leaf, 1 tablespoon of olive oil, and some fresh sage. Simmer for 15 minutes, strain into mugs, and enjoy.

• Italians like to taste their pasta. So don't overload this inherently healthy dish with fatty sauces or toppings. "Use marinara sauce (a meatless tomato sauce) rather than heavy meat sauces and cheeses," advises Dr. Anderson. Or toss with lightly steamed vegetables—broccoli, zucchini, red peppers— and fresh basil, and add a little Parmesan for pasta primavera.

• Don't overdo the olive oil. "Olive oil is a fat," stresses Tammy Baker, RD, general manager for the Dairy Council of Arizona and former spokesperson for the American Dietetic Association. "Just because it's a monounsaturated fat doesn't mean you should use a lot of it. Your best bet is to get 30 percent or less of your total calories from fat."

See also Alcohol, Antioxidants, Exercise, Fish, Garlic, Monounsaturated Fat, Olive Oil, Red Wine

Monounsaturated Fat
How the "Good" Fat Can Help

Of all the mixed messages we've received about our health over the years, perhaps none are as confusing as those involving the dreaded "F" word—*fat*. At first, it seemed logical that it was bad for you—after all, what would make you fat other than fat itself? But then, it became clear that carbohydrates and total calories play as much of a role, if not a greater one, in obesity as fat itself.

When it comes to our hearts, fats have presented the same type of confusion. The common knowledge used to be that all fats were artery cloggers and an overall low-fat approach was the way to go. We now know that fat's relationship with the heart is more complex than this, and it's the type of fat that makes a big difference in our overall heart health.

Enter the monounsaturated fats, one of the good fats that can actually be heart protective. "Monounsaturated fats have well-documented cholesterol-lowering effects," says Ann G. Kulze, MD, founder and CEO of Just Wellness, a wellness consulting firm in Mt. Pleasant, South Carolina, and the author of *Dr. Ann's 10-Step Diet*. "Additionally, some monounsaturated fats, such as extra-virgin olive oil, nuts, seeds, and avocados, have been shown to maintain or even slightly raise levels of 'good' HDL cholesterol."

Moreover, when monounsaturated fats are used to replace the bad fats—saturated fat and trans fatty acids—in the diet, their effects can be even greater. "Saturated and trans fats both elevate blood cholesterol, along with other adverse cardiovascular effects like boosting blood platelet stickiness," says Dr. Kulze. "It is estimated that about 80 percent of the dietary effect on blood cholesterol is derived from ingesting these two fats. And to add insult to injury, trans fats also lower HDL and have been associated with a smaller particle size of 'bad' LDL cholesterol. It is the smaller, dense LDL particles that pose the greatest risk for cardiovascular disease."

So, as you can easily see, if you were to replace any crackers or chips loaded with trans fats (often listed on labels as "partially hydrogenated oils") with healthy snacks like nuts or olives, you not only will be removing a heart hurter from your diet, you also will be adding a heart helper. Talk about a heart-healthy one-two punch!

Of course, experts advise that too much of any type of fat is not a good thing. And since most dietary sources of monounsaturated fat are very calorie dense, they can still lead to obesity if consumed in large quantities. It's for this reason that the American Heart Association recommends limiting overall fat intake to 25 to 35 percent of your daily calories, with monounsaturated fat making up 15 percent of these calories and saturated fat making up 7 to 10 percent.

These Oils Foil Blood Fats

Study after study points to monounsaturated fat's cholesterol-pounding power. In Spain, researchers put 78 men and women on a diet enriched with sunflower oil. After 12 weeks, the participants switched to an olive oil–based diet. Total cholesterol hadn't budged in the men after an additional 4 months and had increased 9 percent in the women, who followed the diet for 7 months. But there was a significant change: The olive oil plan increased HDL levels—by 17 percent in the men and 30 percent in the women.

In another study, researchers in Israel put 17 young men on one of two diets. The first group followed a diet rich in monounsaturated fat (olive oil, avocados, and almonds). The second group consumed a carbohydrate-based diet. Both diets contained similar levels of saturated and polyunsaturated fats. After 3 months, the men consuming the mono-rich diet switched to the carbohydrate plan, and vice versa.

After another 90 days, the researchers tested the men's blood cholesterol. The findings? When the men followed the mono-rich diet, their total cholesterol levels fell by nearly 8 percent, and their LDL levels plunged about

Heart-Healthy Indulgences

Olives: Keep Your Heart Young

Want to hold off Father Time for a while and lower cholesterol as well? Start enjoying olives, which are tasty treats that can do both.

Olives get a big health bonus from where olive trees grow—the sunny climes of California and the Mediterranean region. Blazing sunshine produces a bounty of anthocyanins, flavonoids, and phenols, natural plant substances that fight oxidation caused by the sun's ultraviolet light. Inside your body, these phytochemicals fight the oxidation that may cause aging.

Like the oil they produce, olives are rich in monounsaturated fat, which helps clobber cholesterol and reduce blood clotting, another risk factor for heart disease. As a bonus, monounsaturated oil may also offer some protection against breast cancer.

Eight large black olives or 10 stuffed green olives have a mere 45 calories and 5 grams of fat. But olives do have one potential drawback: They're salty. A serving of 10 large green olives may contain more than 900 milligrams of salt. For people who are sodium sensitive, putting them at risk for high blood pressure, a healthy sodium limit is 2,400 milligrams a day. So, if you're a huge fan of olives, try to limit other sources of salt in your diet.

To benefit from olives without overindulging, use them in some of your favorite dishes.

- Scatter them on a pizza with no cheese and extra sauce.
- Serve them alongside vegetables, low-fat dip, and zesty cheese.

14 percent. No such beneficial changes occurred while the men were following the carbohydrate-based plan.

More recently, two British studies evaluated the cholesterol-lowering effectiveness of a diet high in monounsaturated fatty acids. One involved healthy middle-aged men, and the other tracked young men with a family history of coronary heart disease. At the end of both studies, total and LDL cholesterol levels were significantly lower in the men who ate the diet high in monounsaturated fats than in those who had the control diet higher in saturated fat. The researchers concluded that diets in which saturated fat is partially replaced by monounsaturated fats can achieve significant reductions in total and LDL cholesterol concentrations, even when the same amount of total fat and calories is consumed.

A study by researchers at Harvard University and Brigham and Women's Hospital in Boston showed that dieters who ate large amounts of monounsaturated fats lost weight. The primary source of monounsaturated fat in the study was peanut butter.

A Fat by Any Other Name

There's no doubt about it: Replacing the saturated fat in your diet with unsaturated oils can do your heart good. But don't go hog wild even with monounsaturated oils, experts advise. "Don't pour them over foods," says Michael Klaper, MD, health director of the Royal Atlantic Health Spa in Pompano Beach, Florida, and author of *Vegan Nutrition: Pure and Simple*. "I generally recommend using a tablespoon or two a day at most."

A small amount of oil can go a long way. You might drizzle a bit of olive oil on a crusty piece of Italian bread for lunch and use the remaining allotment on your salad at dinner. Or lightly coat a skillet with it. "Rather than pouring olive oil in the pan, just brush the bottom with a light coat of oil," suggests Dr. Klaper.

In a nutshell: "Don't increase your intake of monounsaturated fat. Decrease your consumption of saturated fat," advises Evelyn Tribole, RD, a dietitian in Beverly Hills, California, and author of *Healthy Homestyle Cooking*. "And if you pay attention to food labels, it's so easy to cut back."

See also Avocados, Canola Oil, Mediterranean Diet, Nuts, Olive Oil, Polyunsaturated Fat

Niacin

Cholesterol Help from a Simple Supplement

Vitamin supplements have gotten a bad rap of late. Studies have shown that "the big three" antioxidants—vitamins C and E and beta-carotene (which converts into vitamin A)—do not offer much benefit when taken in supplement form.

But there's one vitamin that seems to lower LDL ("bad") cholesterol and triglycerides as well as raise HDL ("good") cholesterol. It's vitamin B_3, otherwise known as niacin. And on top of everything else, niacin costs a lot less than prescription cholesterol-lowering drugs.

Research actually offers a mixed review for niacin. Studies have shown that getting the cholesterol-busting effects of niacin requires a dose of 1,000 to 3,000 milligrams a day. That's much higher than the Daily Value of niacin, and levels this high can only be prescribed by a doctor.

In addition, a 1994 study showed that high levels of niacin can cause serious liver side effects. However, those researchers used higher-than-recommended doses. More recent research has shown that proper doses lead to infrequent liver complications. Still, if your doctor prescribes niacin, he or she will monitor your liver enzymes so that the dose can be modified or discontinued at the first sign of any trouble. Other side effects of niacin may include gout and high blood sugar, so it may not be prescribed if you have high uric acid levels (which cause gout) or diabetes.

The other big reason doctors have snubbed niacin is its most common side effect. People who take it often experience flushing, similar to a hot flash. It's like a mild sunburn that usually occurs on the face and sometimes on the chest. This unpleasant effect usually subsides as your body gets used to the drug. Research shows that flushing can be eliminated 80 percent of the time by taking niacin with meals; avoiding alcohol, spicy foods, and hot liquids; and not skipping doses. It may also help to take an aspirin before the niacin.

Whether niacin in supplement form is right for you depends on your cholesterol profile. Never start taking large doses of niacin on your own. Instead, check with your doctor.

Nuts

A Handful of Health

As prescription drugs like statins are becoming more and more effective at lowering cholesterol—and more and more doctors are prescribing them—it may sometimes seem as if good nutrition is losing the fight against cholesterol.

That's why study results such as these are so exciting: Researchers at the University of Toronto were able to lower levels of LDL cholesterol by 35 percent through diet alone—which is a bigger drop than even people taking statin drugs typically see. The other good news? A large component of the diet used by the University of Toronto researchers was delicious, heart-healthy almonds.

The diet, known as the Portfolio Eating Plan, has created quite a buzz in the medical community recently. In four different studies published between 2002 and 2006, the researchers showed that a vegetarian diet consisting of soy, plant sterols, and viscous fiber from plentiful fruits and vegetables could consistently match the cholesterol-lowering benefits of drugs in almost 200 men and women with high cholesterol. One key component of the Portfolio Eating Plan is 30 grams of almonds every day.

Take a closer look at almonds, and it's easy to see why they have heart researchers so excited. They're one of the best sources of monounsaturated fats around. Almost three-quarters of the fat in almonds (72 percent) is monounsaturated, which has been shown to lower total and "bad" LDL cholesterol without detrimentally affecting the "good" HDL cholesterol. Plus, 21 percent is the nearly equally healthy polyunsaturated fat, and only a minuscule 7 percent is unhealthy saturated fat.

Beyond just good fat, almonds provide as much protein as red meat. And let's not forget about their heart-healthy antioxidants either. "Almonds are uniquely high in gamma-tocopherol, a form of vitamin E that seems to play a key role in arterial health," says Ann G. Kulze, MD, founder and CEO of Just Wellness, a wellness consulting firm in Mt. Pleasant, South Carolina, and the author of *Dr. Ann's 10-Step Diet*. In fact, just 1 ounce (or 20 to 25 almonds) provides 35 percent of the Daily Value of vitamin E. Throw in 5 grams, or 20 percent of your Daily Value, of fiber in each serving of almonds, and you have a food that fights cholesterol on multiple levels.

A Mixed Bag of Goodness

Now before you get too excited about almonds, keep in mind that most other nuts are good for your heart as well. Walnuts, in particular, boast almost as much healthy polyunsaturated fat as almonds do monounsaturated fat. In fact, 70 percent of the fat in walnuts is polyunsaturated, and their ratio of polyunsaturated fat to saturated fat is 7 to 1.

What's more, walnuts don't just have any ordinary polyunsaturated fat. "Walnuts, especially English walnuts, have a cardiovascular edge because of their high omega-3 fat content," says Dr. Kulze. That's right—the same type of fats that make cold-water fish such a heart-smart choice are also found in abundance in walnuts.

Of course, a can of mixed nuts may have almost as many benefits as almonds or walnuts. "Nuts are one of the richest sources of monounsaturated fats around," says Christopher Gardner, PhD, of the Stanford Prevention Research Center at Stanford University Medical Center. And when you throw into the mix the magnesium, copper, folate, protein, potassium, fiber, and vitamin E found in nuts, what you get is a plethora of heart-healthy benefits. There's also the curious Brazil nut, which can provide eight times the Daily Value of the trace mineral and antioxidant selenium in just 1 ounce.

Add it all up, and nuts have a lot of heart-healthy benefits. It's the reason that Ralph Felder, MD, PhD, section chief for cardiovascular nutrition at the Good Samaritan Medical Center in Phoenix and author of *The Bonus Years Diet*, made nuts one of the cornerstone foods of the diet in his book. "Nuts have a high ratio of polyunsaturated and monounsaturated fat to saturated fat, and this leads to decreases in bad cholesterol, or LDL," he says. "However, the decrease in bad cholesterol is greater than would just be predicted by this ratio, so other factors seem to be involved in nuts reducing bad cholesterol. Nuts also contain soluble fiber and phytosterols that prevent cholesterol's absorption. These factors are likely to contribute to the cholesterol-lowering effects of nuts."

Nuts about Research

Even when placed under the scrutiny of scientific study, all of nuts' healthy attributes really seem to shine through. Beyond the pivotal role of almonds in the Portfolio Eating Plan, other research has shown the benefits of nuts. Here's what the researchers have discovered so far.

At Loma Linda University in California, scientists examined the link between eating nuts like almonds, walnuts, and peanuts and a reduced risk of heart disease in more than 31,000 people. The researchers found that those who ate nuts more than four times a week had about half the risk of suffering a heart attack (fatal or nonfatal) of those who ate nuts less than once a week. Twenty-nine percent of the nuts consumed were almonds.

"There are several possible reasons why almonds and other nuts seem to be capable of lowering blood cholesterol levels," says Gary E. Fraser, MD, PhD, professor of medicine at Loma Linda University School of Public Health and head of the study. "Almost certainly, nuts' high level of monounsaturated fat is a major factor. But nuts are also a very good source of an amino acid called arginine, which is a dietary precursor of a chemical called nitric oxide, a major EDRF (endothelium-derived relaxing factor)." This chemical, which is released in the lining of the artery wall, seems to help prevent atherosclerosis, he explains.

Other studies have also offered evidence that nuts can help the heart. A 2004 study examined how walnuts and walnut oil could affect cholesterol levels in 20 men and 3 women who were overweight and had high cholesterol levels. Part of the group was placed on an average American diet, and the other part of the group added an ounce of walnuts and a teaspoon of walnut oil to their diet.

After the conclusion of the study, those who ate the walnut-fortified diet experienced drops in total cholesterol and "bad" LDL cholesterol of 11 to 12 percent. This research is part of the reason that the FDA now allows walnuts to be labeled as a heart-healthy food.

Enjoy in Moderation

Nuts may be good for your heart, but what's often lost in this heart-healthy hubbub is the fact that all types of nuts are extremely fat and calorie dense. In fact, it's almost uncanny how similar different kinds of nuts are in their calorie and fat content. On average, a 1-ounce serving of nuts dishes up around 200 calories, about 70 to 75 percent of which come from fat. And though monounsaturated and polyunsaturated fats are better choices than saturated fat, they can still lead to obesity if you go overboard.

Luckily, Dr. Kulze has a simple tip to avoid eating too many nuts. "Limit consumption to one small handful—or about 1 ounce—every day," she says.

"You can buy great 1-ounce containers to help you accomplish this. Fill them up and take them with you as a super-healthy, portable snack. Also, *never* eat them out of the jar. Just take your 1-ounce portion, close the lid, and put them away."

David L. Katz, MD, MPH, director of the Yale-Griffin Prevention Research Center in Derby, Connecticut, and author of *Dr. David Katz's Flavor-Full Diet*, has another bit of advice when it comes to nuts. Because nuts are so calorie dense, "you have to make room for the calories," he says. "So think about nuts as a dietary substitution, not an addition."

Get Nuts without Going Nuts

A handful of nuts might make the perfect snack, but there are other ways to spice up meals and snacks with them. Here are some suggestions—and a few preparation and storage tips, too.

- To enjoy the flavor of almonds without the added fat or salt of the canned kind, toast the nuts yourself. Here's how: Spread whole raw almonds in a single layer across a shallow pan. Place the pan in a cold oven, then heat to 350°F. Stir the nuts occasionally. When they're lightly toasted (8 to 12 minutes), remove from the pan and cool.

  You can microwave almonds, too. Place ½ cup of raw almonds on a microwave-safe plate or bowl. Then zap the almonds for 2 to 6 minutes on high power, stirring once a minute. Let cool.

- If you hate to crack walnuts, buy the pre-shelled kind. They're just as fresh and flavorful as the unshelled variety. Refrigerate them if you plan to use them within a few months; otherwise, freeze them.

- To get rid of walnuts' sometimes astringent aftertaste, which is caused by the tannin in the nuts' dry, papery skins, drop the nuts in boiling water for a minute or two (a process called blanching). Or simply add walnuts at the end of a recipe.

- Sprinkle your hot or cold cereal, waffles, or pancakes with slivered almonds or other nuts. Or stir ground nuts into fat-free or low-fat yogurt.

- Add chopped walnuts to pancake batter. To further reduce fat and cholesterol, prepare the batter with fat-free milk and egg substitute.

- Toss a small amount of chopped walnuts into a salad.

- Stir chopped or ground almonds or other nuts into cooked vegetables, pasta dishes, soups, and salads.

- Sprinkle chopped, shelled walnuts over steamed brussels sprouts or baked sweet potatoes.

- Replace small amounts of meat, fish, or chicken in main-dish casseroles with ground almonds. You'll boost your consumption of healthier mono-unsaturated fat while you reduce your intake of saturated fat.

- Toss about ½ cup of nuts into homemade bread.

- For a snack, combine almonds and dried dates.

Oats

Redemption for a Cholesterol Superstar

When you see oats on a list of cholesterol-busting foods, your first reaction might be, "Not again!" Most of this consternation stems from oat bran, which in the late 1980s had a meteoric rise and colossal fall as a health food that mirrored that of some teenage pop stars. What began as a mad push to add oat bran to all of our favorite foods ended with a spectacular thud when a study concluded that oat bran lowered cholesterol about as well as white bread.

Though the hype for oat bran was undoubtedly overblown, the unfortunate outcome of the whole thing was that many people turned their backs on oats completely. And oats, whether in oatmeal, bread, cereal, or other foods, are a fantastic cholesterol-dropping food.

You know how oatmeal gets sticky when you cook it? That sticky stuff is the soluble fiber beta-glucan, which actually traps cholesterol in the intestine and shuffles it out of the body. Additionally, oats appear to have other cholesterol fighters: chemical compounds known as saponins. In animal studies, these compounds appear to bind to cholesterol and remove it from the body. They do the same thing to bile acids, which can play a role in causing cholesterol levels to rise.

The other good news about oats is that it doesn't take much to derive the cholesterol-busting benefits of the grain. Studies show that just ¾ cup of dry oatmeal, which cooks up to about 1½ cups, each day can help lower total cholesterol by as much as 5 percent.

The Proof Is in the Porridge

Researchers have conducted a number of studies on the association between consuming oat bran and lower blood cholesterol levels. Investigators at Northwestern University Feinberg School of Medicine in Chicago divided 80 men and women with high cholesterol into two groups. The first group ate two servings (about 2 ounces per serving) of instant oats a day. The second group continued to follow their normal eating habits. After 8 weeks, the oat group's total cholesterol had declined by about 15 milligrams/deciliter (mg/dl).

At the University of Kentucky College of Medicine in Lexington, 20 men with high cholesterol consumed diets supplemented with either oat bran or wheat bran, both of which were added to cereal and muffins. After 3 weeks, the total cholesterol of the men eating oat bran had fallen 12.8 percent, and their "bad" LDL cholesterol had declined 12.1 percent. The men who consumed wheat bran saw no such improvements in cholesterol.

In an attempt to draw conclusions from the existing research on oat bran and cholesterol, researchers from all over the world, including the United States, pooled data from 10 studies and 1,300 people. The researchers found that people who ate 3 grams a day of the soluble fiber found in oat bran (equal to about 1⅓ bowls of oat bran cereal) saw their blood cholesterol fall an average of nearly 6 mg/dl in 3 months or less. What's more, those who began with the highest cholesterol readings (230 mg/dl or more) experienced the greatest decreases in blood cholesterol—an average decline of 16 mg/dl.

Five Ways to Feel Your Oats

Want to add oat bran to your diet? These tips can help.

- Choose a whole oat product with the words *rolled oats, steel-cut oats, Irish oats,* or *oat bran* on the label. Also steer clear of instant oatmeal, which doesn't offer the same benefits as whole oat products.

• Top a bowl of oat bran or oatmeal with a low-fat, low-cholesterol topping such as fat-free milk, fresh fruit, or even a dollop or two of fat-free flavored yogurt.

• Try adding a small amount of oat bran to other dishes, suggests James W. Anderson, MD, professor of medicine and clinical nutrition at the University of Kentucky College of Medicine in Lexington and author of *Dr. Anderson's High-Fiber Fitness Plan.* "You can mix oat bran or oatmeal into ground-meat dishes, casseroles, and pancakes," he says.

• Bake your own oat bran muffins using low-fat ingredients, including fat-free milk, egg substitute, and unsaturated oil instead of butter. Try using ¾ cup of oat bran for every ¼ cup of flour in a 12-muffin recipe. For extra-tasty muffins, try adding a small amount of crushed pineapple to the mix, suggests Dr. Anderson.

• Be wary of store-bought oat bran muffins. "They can contain a lot of fat," says Robert J. Nicolosi, PhD, director of the Cardiovascular Research Center at the University of Lowell in Massachusetts. "The ideal way to get fiber is through grains and cereals."

Don't expect a bowl of oat bran to compensate for a fat-laden diet. "All of the soluble fiber in the world isn't going to compensate for eating too much saturated fat," notes Linda Van Horn, RD, PhD, associate professor of preventive medicine at Northwestern University Feinberg School of Medicine in Chicago.

Olive Oil
The King of Heart-Healthy Oils

When it comes to what you put in your mouth, *oil* is often the equivalent of a bad word in heart-healthy circles. In fact, in the USDA's new Food Guide Pyramid, you'll notice that in addition to the five food groups, there is a tiny sixth sliver that's barely detectable unless you look closely. That sliver is the oils, which, according to the USDA, should be "used sparingly."

But for some reason, there's one oil that gets a pass from all this criticism—olive oil. And when you look into the research behind this ancient oil, you'll understand why it's held above the rest.

The Aura of Olive Oil

In ancient times, the Greek physician Hippocrates praised olive oil as a natural remedy. More than 2,000 years later, the research suggests that Hippocrates knew what he was talking about.

Olive oil is a rich source of monounsaturated fats, which have been shown to lower levels of the "bad" cholesterol (LDL) while maintaining or even slightly raising levels of the "good" (HDL). Of all the fats, monounsaturated ones are the healthiest. Polyunsaturated fats (found in vegetable oil) may lower LDL, but they also lower HDL. Saturated fats (found in butter and coconut oil) tend to raise cholesterol levels. The worst of all may be the trans fatty acids (found in some margarines and shortenings), which raise LDL, lower HDL, and promote smaller LDL particle size, which puts you at a greater risk of heart disease. As you can see, replacing other oils in your diet with olive oil can have some big benefits.

Of course, these oils don't exist in our diets in isolation. The newest research has shown that the ratio of one fat to another can have a big impact on our overall heart health. This makes olive oil even more important than it was previously thought to be. "I prefer olive oil over the polyunsaturated vegetable oils like corn oil, sunflower oil, safflower oil, and soybean oil, because they are slightly less prone to oxidation, and oxidized fats are toxic," says Ann G. Kulze, MD, founder and CEO of Just Wellness, a wellness consulting firm in Mt. Pleasant, South Carolina, and the author of *Dr. Ann's 10-Step Diet*. "In addition, they have a favorable effect on omega-3 and omega-6 ratios. Polyunsaturated vegetable oils are rich in omega-6 fats, and Americans consume too many of them in relation to omega-3s. So when you replace the omega-6 fats with the monounsaturated fats found in olive oil, you're helping to improve the ratio."

If you need any more reason to try olive oil, some cutting-edge research has shown that something heart healthy may be going on in the oil beyond just monounsaturated fat. "Recent clinical research has clearly established that the polyphenols (plant chemicals) in extra-virgin olive oil have very important antioxidant effects in addition to olive oil's effect on the blood lipids," says Ralph Felder, MD, PhD, section chief for cardiovascular nutrition at the Good Samaritan Medical Center in Phoenix and author of *The Bonus Years Diet.* "Tests in actual patients have shown that the anti-oxidant effect of these polyphenols really does protect the blood vessels by promoting the function of the endothelial lining cells." (For more information on the benefits of extra-virgin olive oil, see "Extra-Virgin Olive Oil: Worth the Extra $$$.")

An Olive Oil Primer

Of course, beyond what the research says, it doesn't hurt that olive oil actually tastes great! It's perfect for cooking, for dressing a salad, or for drizzling on delicious bread. But, as with all fats in the diet, you should enjoy olive oil in moderation.

Luckily, olive oil's strong flavor makes even that task easy. "Compared with some other oils, olive oil is so flavorful that you can use less of it," says Barbara Levine, PhD, RD, associate clinical professor of nutrition in medicine at Weill Medical College of Cornell University in New York City.

Olive oil connoisseurs categorize the flavor of olive oil as mild (with a light or buttery taste), semifruity (a stronger, more olivelike flavor), or fruity (with an intense olive flavor). And despite what you may have heard, the color of olive oil has nothing to do with its flavor. Like wine, olive oil gets its unique color, flavor, and aroma from the olives used and the climate and

---

Versions of Virgins

When it comes to olive oil, "refined" isn't a compliment. Confused? Relax: This guide can help you decipher the labels and select the perfect oil.

Extra-virgin olive oil. Produced in limited quantities, extra-virgin oil is the best and most expensive grade of olive oil that money can buy. Most people use extra-virgin oil, which has an intense fruity or peppery flavor, to flavor foods after they've been cooked rather than as a cooking oil.

Virgin olive oil. The flavor of this oil isn't as perfect as that of extra-virgin oil and is slightly more acidic.

Olive oil. Most people use this blend of refined and unrefined virgin oils for cooking.

"Extra-light" olive oil. Perfect for baking, this extra-refined oil has little or no olive taste. But don't be fooled: Light olive oil contains the same amount of fat and calories as other oils.

soil conditions in which they were grown. So you may want to taste-test olive oil to find the variety and brand most pleasing to your palate.

Here's how to get more olive oil into your diet.

• Spread crusty bread with olive oil rather than butter, suggests Dr. Levine. Or rub a toasted slice of bread with a piece of garlic, then drizzle the bread with olive oil.

• Dress salads the Mediterranean way—with a small amount of extra-virgin olive oil and a little bit of vinegar, suggests Gene A. Spiller, DSc,

Heart-Healthy Indulgences

Extra-Virgin Olive Oil: Worth the Extra $$$

Some things in life cost more than others. In the case of extra-virgin olive oil, the added expense is worth it, since studies show that the oil will benefit your health.

Researchers in Spain (where use of olive oil is widespread) asked 24 men to prepare meals with either refined or extra-virgin olive oil. After 3 months, the experts concluded that extra-virgin oil was more effective than regular olive oil at stopping the men's LDL cholesterol from oxidizing. Researchers think that white blood cells pick up only oxidized LDL and deposit it in artery linings; thus, since extra-virgin oil contains high levels of antioxidants, it may help slow plaque formation in the arteries (atherosclerosis).

The good news doesn't stop there. A study in Greece showed that people with the lowest lifetime consumption of extra-virgin olive oil had a 2½ times greater chance of developing rheumatoid arthritis than those with the highest consumption. Rheumatologist Hayes Wilson, MD, spokesperson for the Arthritis Foundation, says, "If you have rheumatoid arthritis in your family and want to take every possible step to protect yourself, you might try adding olive oil to your diet." And, he adds, since the type of oil consumed in Greece is extra-virgin, that may offer additional protection.

Although all the standard grades of olive oil are high in heart-healthy monounsaturated fats, extra-virgin is best because it's made from the first pressing of the olives (with acid levels under 1 percent). The other grades, while still good for you, are generally more acidic and processed.

PhD, director of the Health Research and Studies Center in Los Altos, California, and author of *The Superpyramid Eating Program.*

• Brush corn on the cob with extra-virgin olive oil rather than butter or margarine, suggests Dr. Spiller.

• Add olive oil to sauces, marinades, and any other dish in which you want a more robust flavor, says Tammy Baker, RD, general manager for the Dairy Council of Arizona and former spokesperson for the American Dietetic Association.

• Bathe fresh garlic and spinach with a small amount of olive oil spray and sauté in a nonstick skillet, suggests Lynn Fischer, author of *Healthy Indulgences.* Spinach lovers will enjoy this Sicilian-style dish, she adds.

• Sauté or bake fish in olive oil rather than butter, says Dr. Levine. "Olive oil expands in the pan, so you need much less of it," she says.

• Bake with olive oil. Yes, you read right. "People in Italy bake magnificent desserts with olive oil," says Dr. Levine. "You can substitute olive oil for butter, margarine, or vegetable shortening in cakes, pies, and other desserts." She suggests using a light variety, so you won't taste olive oil in your dessert.

Avoid cooking with extra-virgin olive oil, advises Dr. Levine. "Heating this oil will accomplish only what's called perfuming the kitchen," she says. "That is, the olive oil goes into the air rather than into the food. Save extra-virgin oil for salads or for drizzling over pasta."

Before You Get All Oiled Up

Don't forget that olive oil is still 100 percent fat and contains 120 calories per tablespoon. So overusing olive oil may cause you to gain weight—not a heart-smart move, say experts.

"Many people are drowning their foods in olive oil, thinking that they're doing themselves a service," says Karen Miller Kovach, RD, chief nutritionist at Weight Watchers International in Jericho, New York. But it's better to substitute olive oil for saturated fats such as butter, says Kovach, than to add olive oil to an already high-fat diet.

Dr. Levine agrees. "Don't consume lots of olive oil or any other kind of oil. Anoint your food with a small amount of olive oil, like the Italians do."

See also Mediterranean Diet

Oranges

A Ray of Sunshine for Your Heart

By now, it's well established that fruits and vegetables of all varieties are heart healthy. This is one of the main reasons the government recently upped its daily fruit and vegetable recommendation from five a day to a whopping nine.

But oranges, aside from just generally being delicious, may offer some specific benefits to the heart. What's more, research seems to indicate that multiple parts of the fruit, from the peel to the juice, can benefit the heart in different ways.

Some of the first research done specifically about oranges and heart health had to do with the juice. At the University of Western Ontario in London, Canada, researchers looked at the effects of different amounts of orange juice on the cholesterol levels of 25 men and women with high cholesterol. After 4 weeks of drinking three glasses of orange juice a day, the study participants' levels of "bad" LDL cholesterol dropped by 16 percent and their levels of "good" HDL cholesterol rose by 21 percent.

At 110 calories per 8-ounce glass of orange juice, though, it may not be realistic to drink that much every day. Moreover, this relatively small study still leaves in question exactly how much juice would really be helpful for cholesterol levels over the long run.

Luckily, research has shown that oranges can help your heart in other ways, too. Oranges are well known for their high vitamin C content, and they are also good sources of fiber, folate, potassium, and calcium, among other vitamins and minerals. But one of the most powerful cholesterol fighters in oranges may be the lesser-known polymethoxylated flavones, or PMFs, which are a group of flavonoids found in the highest concentrations in orange and tangerine peels. Some experts believe that these powerful flavonoids work by inhibiting the synthesis of cholesterol and triglycerides in the liver.

Human tests on the effects of PMFs on cholesterol levels are currently under way, and the results were quite promising in animal tests. Hamsters that were fed a diet containing 1 percent PMFs experienced drops in LDL cholesterol of 32 to 40 percent. No effects were noted on HDL cholesterol, however.

If you're interested in trying PMFs as a potential cholesterol fighter, a supplement called Sytrinol is available that contains almost 20 times the flavonoids of the average glass of orange juice. Of course, including good old oranges, orange juice, and various other citrus fruits among your "daily nine" will provide a number of healthy benefits, potentially lowering your cholesterol being just one of them.

Pectin
The Fiber King

It's no surprise that you should eat more fiber to keep cholesterol levels at bay. Fiber is the main reason that the American Heart Association recently revised their dietary guidelines to focus more on fruits, vegetables, and whole grains.

But what you may not know is that research has shown that some types of fiber may have a slight advantage over others. One that has done particularly well in studies is pectin, which is found in many fruits and vegetables.

"Like other types of soluble fiber, pectin has the capacity to reduce blood cholesterol levels," says Thomas Bersot, MD, PhD, clinical professor of medicine at the University of California, San Francisco. "Pectin may interfere with the body's absorption of cholesterol, which helps lower blood cholesterol levels."

But pectin may have another cholesterol-lowering card up its sleeve. It may affect certain enzymes in the liver that produce cholesterol. Here's what the research has shown about pectin.

Staging a Plaque Attack

In a recent study at the Northwest Lipid Research Clinic in Seattle, people with mild to moderate high cholesterol were assigned to receive either a dietary supplement containing pectin and other forms of fiber or a placebo (an inactive pill) for 15 weeks. After that period, all of the participants received the fiber supplement for an additional 36 weeks.

At the end of the trial, researchers noted that both groups had significant, sustained reductions in their levels of "bad" LDL cholesterol. At the same time, they maintained their levels of triglycerides and "good" HDL cholesterol. The decreases in LDL cholesterol, total cholesterol, and the LDL-to-HDL ratio were also greater among those in the group taking the fiber supplement the entire time.

Despite this evidence, Alicia Moag-Stahlberg, RD, a dietitian with Action for Healthy Kids, a nonprofit organization located in Chicago whose mission is to improve children's nutrition and physical activity, does not recommend relying on a supplement alone for your daily intake of fiber. "Try to get your fiber from foods rather than from supplements," she explains. "The supplements lack other nutrients found in fiber-rich foods. Fruits and vegetables contain antioxidants, for example, which may help prevent heart disease and cancer."

Getting Your Peck of Pectin

Keeping this in mind, here are a few quick, simple ways to add more pectin to your diet through foods.

• Load up on fruits and veggies. Pectin-rich fruits include grapefruit, oranges, bananas, strawberries, peaches, apples, grapes, and plums. Pectin-rich vegetables include carrots, lettuce, spinach, beets, brussels sprouts, cabbage, potatoes, onions, and peas.

• Eat more grapefruit. Whether red, white, or pink, grapefruit is one of the best sources of pectin around, and it's also rich in vitamin C.

• Eat the whole fruit or vegetable rather than drink its juice, suggests Martin Yadrick, RD, a dietitian in Manhattan Beach, California, and a spokesperson for the American Dietetic Association. "Juice doesn't contain as much fiber as the fruit itself," he says. Bonus: You'll most likely feel more satisfied after eating a grapefruit or an apple than after downing a glass of juice.

See also Apples

Peppers

One Bright and Bold Cholesterol Cutter

If you're looking for the "deeply colored" fruits and vegetables that the American Heart Association recommends, you can't get much deeper and brighter than the pepper family. These bright colors come with a lot of heart-healthy benefits: Deeper colors generally equal a greater amount of antioxidants, according to Christopher Gardner, PhD, of the Stanford Prevention Research Center at Stanford University Medical Center. The bold reds, oranges, yellows, greens, and even purples and browns of bell peppers are positively packed with these nutrients.

Though bell peppers vary in color, they are technically all the same plant, *Capsicum annuum*, which, along with tomatoes and eggplant, is a member of the nightshade family. As the same plant, all bell peppers have similar levels of some heart-healthy nutrients, most notably three times the Daily Value of vitamin C, one dose of the Daily Value of vitamin A, as well as healthy amounts of vitamin B_6, fiber, and numerous other nutrients. All of this in a vegetable that is delicious with almost any dish and contains just 24 calories per 1-cup serving!

Recent research, however, has shown that different-colored bell peppers may have varying levels of antioxidant potential. In 2007, researchers at Louisiana State University looked at the antioxidant content of green, yellow, orange, and red peppers. They discovered that the red pepper had the highest levels of antioxidants, while the green pepper had the lowest, with the yellow and orange falling somewhere in between. Despite this, the researchers were quick to point out that any of the peppers is still an excellent food choice: All four peppers showed significant abilities to prevent the oxidation of cholesterol during the study.

The Chile Choice

Based on this research, we know that sweet bell peppers are at best a great cholesterol fighter and at worst a very healthy food choice. But what's interesting about peppers is that another variety, the chile pepper, may fight cholesterol in a completely different fashion.

Undoubtedly, a certain percentage of the population gets a real kick from eating the spicy, five-alarm soups, stews, salsas, sauces, and various other dishes created with chile peppers. As it turns out, those folks are doing more for their health than just building up an immunity to spicy foods. Like their milder, sweeter cousins the bell peppers, chile peppers are a rich source of both vitamin A and vitamin C, but they have an extra ingredient as well: capsaicin. This substance, which gives the peppers their punch, may lower triglycerides, a type of blood fat that is a risk factor for heart disease. In addition, chile peppers may help the body break down dangerous clots, further reducing your risk of heart attack and stroke. Here's what the studies have shown about chile peppers.

The Science Behind Smokin' Hot Peppers

A number of animal studies have examined the effects of capsaicin on blood cholesterol and other types of blood fats. A several-decades-old study of rabbits showed that introducing capsaicin to a high-cholesterol diet over a period of 5 weeks reduced levels of total cholesterol and triglycerides and improved the ratio of total cholesterol to "good" HDL cholesterol. In more recent studies involving rats, however, capsaicin had a significant impact on triglyceride levels but not on cholesterol. Yet another study of rats showed that capsaicin may prevent the oxidation of cholesterol, which is the process that causes cholesterol to deposit itself on the arterial walls and ultimately lead to heart disease.

As you can see, studies have been sending us some mixed messages on the potency of peppers. But even if the capsaicin in peppers just lowers triglycerides, which most studies seem to agree on, it still plays an important role in reducing heart disease. What's more, other studies suggest that adding hot peppers to your diet may help you boost metabolism and in turn lose more weight. And weight loss is another important factor in keeping cholesterol levels under control.

Add Some Heat to Your Meals

Bell peppers are among the most versatile vegetables and are easy to include in your meals. Think of almost any recipe—from soups and sauces to salads and entrées—and bell peppers will more than likely be an ingredient. Chile peppers, however, are usually reserved for those dishes that require some bite. Here are some tips for spicing up your life a little more with chiles as well as some practical advice for avoiding the burn.

• Add a small amount of hot peppers to your salads to give them an extra spiciness.

• Throw chile peppers into your homemade chili.

• Try chopped or ground chile peppers in homemade bread to add a little flair.

• If you're new to chile peppers, err on the side of caution at first. It's always easier to add more spice than it is to take it back out once it's in.

• Chile peppers can burn more than your mouth, so wear protective gloves when handling them and always wash your hands afterward. It's also a good idea not to inhale the fumes directly.

• If you are feeling the burn, wash the peppers down with milk instead of water. Milk contains a protein called casein that coats the mouth and smothers capsaicin's flames. Rice, bananas, or bread can also put out the fire in a pinch.

See also Weight Loss

Plant Stanols and Sterols

The "Secret Ingredients" in Plants

Margarine is hardly what most people consider a health food. And when researchers learned more about the risks of trans fatty acids that are common in hard stick margarines—namely higher "bad" LDL cholesterol levels, lower "good" HDL cholesterol levels, and an increased risk of heart attack—this became even more true.

Then in 1995, a Finnish company called the Raisio Group introduced the margarine Benecol to the world. And, quite contrary to the conventional wisdom of the day, this margarine claimed that it could actually *lower* LDL and total cholesterol levels. Subsequent studies showed that it could do just that—doses of 1 to 3 grams of Benecol daily decreased LDL cholesterol by 6 to 15 percent.

How did a group of Finns turn a seemingly unhealthy food into a healthy one? The secret, it turns out, is a plant compound known as a stanol. Specifically, the active ingredient in Benecol is "plant stanol ester." A 1-tablespoon serving of the spread provides almost 1 gram of plant stanol esters and half a gram of plant stanols. (The National Cholesterol Education Program has said that 2 grams of stanols a day can be heart protective.) Stanols, along with their plant compound cousins, sterols, fight cholesterol in a way that's different than most of the other foods on our heart-healthy list.

Throughout this book, when we talk about something *fighting* cholesterol, it's usually just a convenient metaphor. But in the case of plant stanols and sterols, they are quite literally fighting with cholesterol for absorption in the body. "Stanols and sterols are cholesterol-like plant compounds," says David L. Katz, MD, MPH, director of the Yale-Griffin Prevention Research Center in Derby, Connecticut, and author of *Dr. David Katz's Flavor-Full Diet*. "They compete with cholesterol for absorption in the bloodstream and cause more of it to leave the body through the intestines."

The Straight Scoop

Despite all the recent buzz about them, plant stanols and sterols are nothing new. They're compounds that are common in foods that we've been eating for years. "Sesame oil, flaxseeds, rice bran oil, wheat germ, sunflower seeds, nuts, soybeans, and avocados are the richest sources," says Ann G. Kulze, MD, founder and CEO of Just Wellness, a wellness consulting firm in Mt. Pleasant, South Carolina, and the author of *Dr. Ann's 10-Step Diet*. Studies have shown that leafy green vegetables are also a rich source of sterols.

Considering how common these compounds are in our diets, you might be wondering why we've only been hearing about them over the last few years. The main reason for this is that it takes large doses of stanols and sterols to make an impact on blood pressure—at least larger than foods alone can provide. "The only way to get significant amounts of stanols and sterols is from specially formulated spreads, such as Benecol, or supplements," says Dr. Katz.

Despite this, Dr. Kulze says that you can still derive some value from eating foods rich in stanols and sterols. Here's what all the research has shown on the topic.

Spreading the Word

In recent years, a number of landmark studies have shown the positive effects of specific, targeted diets on lowering cholesterol. One common element among these diets is the inclusion of plant sterols.

One of the most remarkable and well developed of these diets is the Portfolio Eating Plan, an eating regimen devised by researchers at the University of Toronto in 2002. The diet was originally vegetarian in nature, and it was built mainly around foods such as almonds; soy proteins; oats, barley, and other high-fiber foods; abundant fruits and vegetables; and, of course, margarine with plant sterols.

Since 2002, almost 200 men and women with high cholesterol have been subjected to slightly different versions of the diet in four separate clinical trials. Across the board, the positive results of the diet on blood cholesterol levels have been dramatic. Perhaps most impressive was study number two of the Portfolio Eating Plan, in which participants experienced an average drop of 35 percent in their levels of "bad" LDL cholesterol. What's more, this drop occurred after just 2 weeks on the diet, a result that rivals the effectiveness of statin drugs for lowering cholesterol. In fact, in a separate study of the Portfolio Eating Plan that directly compared how the diet and statins affected LDL cholesterol levels, the statins lowered LDL 30.9 percent over a 4-week period, and the Portfolio Eating Plan lowered LDL 28.6 percent.

The most recent study of the Portfolio Eating Plan, in 2006, showed that the diet did not need to be entirely vegan, or even vegetarian, to be effective at lowering cholesterol. For this version of the diet, researchers put only four restrictions on participants: For every 1,000 calories consumed, they must eat 1 gram of plant sterols, 22.5 grams of soy protein, 10 grams of viscous fiber (things like oat bran bread, psyllium, and raw eggplant), and 23 grams of almonds.

Other than that, the 55 men and women on the diet could make their own food choices, be they vegetarian or not. Even with this additional freedom, patients lowered their LDL levels by 20 percent.

The Portfolio Eating Plan isn't the only scientifically approved, cholesterol-lowering diet that uses stanols and sterols as food staples. Christopher Gardner, PhD, of the Stanford Prevention Research Center at Stanford University Medical Center and his colleagues recently compared the effects of two diets on cholesterol levels among 120 men and women with high cholesterol. One of the diets was a standard American "low-fat" diet, complete with low-fat snacks, low-fat dairy products, low-fat dressings, and various other reduced-fat convenience foods. The other diet was primarily plant-based, and it included abundant fruits, vegetables, whole grains, soy, beans, nuts, and—of course—plant sterols.

After 4 weeks, the sterol-based diet yet again won out. This time, the 59 men and women who followed the vegetarian-style diet saw their total cholesterol drop by an average of 18 points and their LDL drop by 14 points. The 61 folks on the standard "American" low-fat diet dropped 9 and 7 points, respectively.

Good news about stanols and sterols has cropped up in other smaller studies as well. According to Dr. Kulze, a rich source of plant sterols is rice bran oil, a cooking oil more commonly used in Japan and India but available in many specialty stores in the United States. A recent small study of 14 people with high cholesterol showed that rice bran oil lowered LDL cholesterol over a 5-week period when used in place of peanut oil, olive oil, corn oil, canola oil, palm oil, and butter. Despite these encouraging results, researchers were quick to point out that it's still too early to recommend switching to rice bran oil on a massive scale.

A Heart-Healthy Ingredient

These and multiple other studies about stanols and sterols have proven so promising that in September 2000 the FDA allowed manufacturers of foods containing plant sterol or plant stanol ethers to include a heart-health claim on their products. The result has been a virtual explosion of foods containing stanols and sterols, including not only margarine spreads but also mayonnaise, yogurt, cheese, cereal, and bread, among others.

With all these foods claiming to have heart-healthy, cholesterol-lowering benefits, it's best to stick to the FDA's recommendations on stanols and sterols: 1.3 grams of plant sterol esters and 3.4 grams of plant stanol esters are the amounts that have been shown to be heart healthy. It's for this reason that foods must have half that amount—0.65 gram of sterols and 1.7 grams of stanols—to qualify for their heart-health claim.

Just to put this in perspective with a common food, you'd need to eat four servings, or 4 tablespoons, of Benecol spread to get the recommended 3.4 grams of plant stanol esters daily. The makers of Benecol recommend using Benecol Light if you plan to eat that much. Benecol also makes a chewable supplement that provides the recommended 3.4 grams of plant stanol esters in four chews. Benecol recommends taking two chews, twice per day, along with food for best results.

Policosanol
Solve Cholesterol Woes with . . . Wax?

Policosanol is a supplement that has followed an interesting path to prominence. In fact, its rise in stature is not unlike a famous rock band replacing its lead singer with a relatively unknown musician.

In the late 1990s, Cholestin was one of the most popular and effective cholesterol-lowering dietary supplements available on the market. In fact, when the supplement was first studied in the United States, the 83 participants who took Cholestin experienced a 16 percent average decrease in their total cholesterol levels over a 12-week period.

Unfortunately, Cholestin's active ingredient, red yeast rice extract, performed similarly to the active ingredient in the prescription cholesterol-lowering drug lovastatin, which is sold under the brand name Mevacor. To make a long story short, the makers of Mevacor took the makers of Cholestin to court, and the court ruled in 2001 that supplements containing red yeast rice extract could not be sold without a prescription.

Rather than close up shop, though, its makers put a new version of Cholestin on the market that replaced red yeast rice extract with a previously unknown cholesterol-lowering supplement—policosanol. And just like that, the supplement became a cholesterol-cutting superstar.

The Power of Policosanol

As surprising as it sounds, policosanol is actually derived from wax. Though it's relatively new here in the United States, it has been known about and studied in Cuba since the early 1900s. The policosanol developed in Cuba has traditionally been made from sugarcane wax, but the kind used in America comes from beeswax.

Researchers aren't exactly sure how policosanol lowers blood cholesterol levels, but one theory is that it inhibits the synthesis, or formation, of cholesterol in the first place. It also appears to have antioxidant properties that prevent "bad" LDL cholesterol from oxidizing and damaging the arterial walls. Some studies have also indicated that policosanol may reduce blood clot formation in the arteries and improve the flow of blood through the body, but more research is needed in this area.

Though the reasons that policosanol works so well are still a bit hazy, in studies it not only lowers LDL cholesterol significantly but also appears to raise "good" HDL cholesterol. Here's what the research has shown so far.

A Wax That Wows

Despite its relative obscurity, policosanol's effects on cholesterol have been studied extensively—more than 3,000 subjects have taken part in policosanol research to date. One of the most recent trials compared policosanol to the cholesterol-lowering drug atorvastatin in 75 elderly patients with high cholesterol. The subjects were divided into two groups, each of which took a 10-milligram tablet of policosanol or atorvastatin once daily with their evening meal.

The policosanol didn't quite keep pace with the atorvastatin—but it was pretty close. The prescription statin drug lowered LDL cholesterol 28.4 percent and 29.8 percent at 4 and 8 weeks, respectively. But the policosanol wasn't that far behind, lowering cholesterol 17.5 percent after 4 weeks and 23.1 percent after 8 weeks. What's more, the policosanol raised levels of HDL cholesterol by 5.3 percent—an effect that the statin could not duplicate. Both the statin drug and the policosanol also lowered triglyceride levels in the study subjects.

Despite the positive results of this and numerous other studies, some recent research has shed doubt on the effectiveness of policosanol, with little change noted in cholesterol levels in people with moderately high cholesterol levels. But a review of dietary supplements and their effectiveness in preventing coronary artery disease (published by the *Journal of Alternative and Complementary Medicine* in 2007) pointed out that policosanol had far more evidence supporting its use as a treatment for high cholesterol than any other supplement.

Be Supplement Savvy

Though the research on policosanol has undoubtedly been a mixed bag, almost every study done on the supplement has indicated that it is safe, with only a few rare adverse side effects, including upset stomach, diarrhea, headache, skin rash, excess urination, insomnia, and weight loss. Policosanol is also a mild blood-thinning agent, so you may want to steer clear of taking the supplement with other medications that have similar effects, such as aspirin, heparin, warfarin, and clopidogrel. That being said, if the safety of other cholesterol-lowering supplements is a concern, you may want to give policosanol a try, after talking with your doctor about it, of course.

A typical dose of policosanol ranges from 5 milligrams to 20 milligrams daily in capsule form. It should be taken with the evening meal for maximum effectiveness, as evidence has suggested that most cholesterol creation occurs at night. Studies on policosanol have shown that the effectiveness increases with the size of the daily dosage. (In several 6-month trials, 10 milligrams of policosanol a day dropped LDL by an average of 20 to 25 percent; 20 milligrams a day dropped LDL by 25 to 30 percent. Still, it's best to stay within the 20-milligram-a-day window.)

As you may have noticed, the overall dosage of policosanol is fairly small when compared to other supplements. This is another advantage of policosanol, as it makes it a great supplement to take with other potential cholesterol fighters, such as fish oil, garlic, and coenzyme Q_{10}. Together, all these heart-healthy supplements can have an even greater benefit on your overall cholesterol levels.

Polyunsaturated Fat
The "Second Fiddle" of Fats

While the monounsaturated fats found in nuts, olives, olive oil, canola oil, and avocados may be the best choice for fats, they are by no means the only healthy choice. Polyunsaturated fats can also play a role in lowering cholesterol, especially when used in the diet to replace unhealthy saturated fat and trans fatty acids. This is the main reason that the American Heart Association recently revamped their dietary guidelines. They now recommend that 25 to 35 percent of your total daily calories should come from fat—and the majority of those should be monounsaturated or polyunsaturated sources.

The other good news about polyunsaturated fats is that you'll find them in much more abundance than monounsaturated fats. While the foods mentioned above—along with a few seeds—are good sources of "monos," you'll find "polys" in a host of foods we eat every day: corn oil, sunflower oil, sesame oil, fish, as well as nuts and seeds. In addition, the heralded omega-3 fatty acids that you hear so much about are polyunsaturated fats, and they have additional heart-healthy benefits, including lowering blood pressure, preventing clot formation, and preserving the function of blood vessels.

With all this great news, you might wonder why we're calling polyunsaturated fats "second fiddle" to monounsaturated fats. There's a simple reason, actually. "Numerous studies have shown that monounsaturated fats lower LDL cholesterol (the 'bad' kind) while preserving HDL (the 'good' kind), but polyunsaturated fats tend to lower both," says David L. Katz, MD, MPH, director of the Yale-Griffin Prevention Research Center in Derby, Connecticut, and author of *Dr. David Katz's Flavor-Full Diet*. "In addition, not all polyunsaturated fats are created equal. Omega-3s are polyunsaturated fats and are uniquely beneficial, but there are some concerns about an excess of omega-6 fats." (For more information, as well as good choices for polyunsaturated fats, see "All Polys Are Not Created Equal" on page 142.)

Despite these concerns, most heart experts agree that replacing saturated fats and trans fats with *any* type of unsaturated fat is beneficial.

"If you replace the saturated fat you get from animal products—such as meat and dairy foods—with unsaturated fat from plants and vegetables,

All Polys Are Not Created Equal

Some oils with polyunsaturated fats, such as soybean, safflower, grapeseed, and corn oils, contain omega-6 fatty acids, which can hinder the benefits of omega-3s when consumed in excess. Your best bet is to use them sparingly and focus on oils high in monounsaturated fats and omega-3s, along with varying amounts of vitamin E (an antioxidant that is also considered beneficial to heart health).

Oils	Monounsaturates (%)	Polyunsaturates (%)	Saturates (%)	Omega-3 Fatty Acids (%)
Top Choices				
Hazelnut	82	10	8	0
Olive	77	9	14	0.6
Canola	62	31	7	9.7
Peanut	48	34	18	0
Sesame	42	43	15	0.3
Walnut	24	66	10	10.9
Flaxseed	21	68	11	55.8
Use Occasionally*				
Corn	25	62	13	0.7
Soybean	24	61	15	7.1
Grapeseed	17	73	10	0.1
Avoid				
Coconut	6	2	92	0

Source: USDA Nutrient Database

*Safflower and sunflower oils should also be used only occasionally, but actual values vary from manufacturer to manufacturer. Check labels for nutrition information.

you'll be in good shape," says Christopher Gardner, PhD, of the Stanford Prevention Research Center at Stanford University Medical Center, who did a comprehensive review of research comparing monounsaturated and polyunsaturated fat and their relative effects on cholesterol levels. "When it comes to HDL and LDL cholesterol levels, it doesn't matter whether the fats are monounsaturated or polyunsaturated, as long as they're not saturated."

See also Canola Oil, Fish, Fish Oil Supplements, Monounsaturated Fat, Olive Oil

Pomegranates

The Exotic New "Super-Fruit"

When it comes to the media buzz about heart health, pomegranate juice may be this generation's red wine. It has received so much attention in the press lately that this formerly exotic fruit is gradually becoming mainstream. When you cut through the chatter and look at the hard science behind pomegranates, it's easy to understand the excitement.

For those unfamiliar with this exotic newcomer, pomegranates are about the size of a large orange, and they contain hundreds of seeds in a juicy red pulp. This pulp is where pomegranate juice comes from.

Like many fruits and vegetables, pomegranates are rich in antioxidant compounds, including flavonoids. But what sets pomegranates apart is the amount of antioxidants they hold—several times more than most fruits and vegetables. Specifically, pomegranates are rich in polyphenols, the same types of flavonoids found in other proven cholesterol cutters such as green tea and dark chocolate. Pomegranates have been used in the Middle East, Iran, and India as a folk remedy for quite some time.

The Power of Poms

Scientific research on pomegranate juice seems to support the power of its "super-antioxidant" status. Israeli researchers analyzing both human and animal studies estimated that drinking 2 to 3 ounces of pomegranate juice every day for 2 weeks slowed the cholesterol oxidation process—which eventually leads to heart disease—by as much as 40 percent. More recently, Iranian researchers saw significant reductions in "bad" LDL and total cholesterol when they gave pomegranate juice to 22 patients with high cholesterol and diabetes for 8 weeks.

Picking Pomegranates

If you're ready to try the healing power of pomegranates, you have a couple of options. Fresh pomegranates are delicious, but tearing open the fruit, discarding the white membrane, and eating all of those pulp-covered seeds can be messy and time consuming. A better option is pomegranate juice, which is available from a number of companies, including Pom Wonderful (www.PomWonderful.com). Pom Wonderful also just released a pomegranate supplement, which offers the benefits of pomegranates in capsule form. You may want to speak with your doctor before adding this supplement to your regimen, however.

Popcorn

Make It Right for Your Heart

In the world of snack foods, popcorn is truly an enigma. Prepared one way, a cup of popcorn has 31 calories, 0.3 gram of fat, 1.2 grams of fiber, and even 1 gram of protein. If it's prepared another way, though, those numbers blow up like the kernels themselves: A small bag contains 20 grams of fat, 14 of which are saturated. And that's without including the butter topping, which is loaded with bad-for-your-heart trans fatty acids. Throw the butter topping on a large bag of that corn, and now you're talking almost 130 grams of fat, or more than 4 days' worth. No kidding.

This unpleasant comparison is the difference between plain air-popped popcorn and popcorn from your local movie theater. (For more reasons why you should skip the movie popcorn, see "Pass on Movie Popcorn.") As you can see, the method of preparation makes a big difference in popcorn's heart-healthy content.

If you need more reasons to invest in an air popper, consider this. Few snacks can make you feel full with fewer calories than popcorn. This is due in large part to popcorn's high dose of insoluble fiber. Although this type of fiber may not be as beneficial to cholesterol levels as soluble fiber, it still plays a role in your overall heart health. "Insoluble fiber may have cholesterol-lowering effects, albeit not directly like soluble fiber," says Ann G. Kulze, MD, founder and CEO of Just Wellness, a wellness consulting firm in Mt. Pleasant, South Carolina, and the author of *Dr. Ann's 10-Step Diet*. "Insoluble fiber may improve cholesterol metabolism by enhancing insulin sensitivity.

Insulin resistance, the opposite of insulin sensitivity, is associated with elevated LDL cholesterol and reduced HDL levels."

Now, you also may be wondering about the most easily accessible kind of popcorn out there—the microwave kind. Though microwave popcorn manufacturers have met our health demands with dozens of low-fat varieties, experts still recommend approaching these with caution. They need some oil to make them pop, so they'll never be as healthy as the air-popped variety. Plus, air-popped corn gives you more control over the oil, fat, and flavoring content of your popcorn.

Flavor without Fat

Here's how to make home-popped popcorn extra delicious and how to select heart-smart microwaveable or ready-to-eat popcorn.

• To add pizzazz to air-popped corn, lightly spray it with a vegetable oil cooking spray, such as Pam, and get creative with the seasonings by sprinkling the corn with low-fat cheese, or even caraway or mustard seeds.

Pass on Movie Popcorn

If you're like a lot of people, watching the latest blockbuster without a big tub of buttered popcorn is just about unthinkable. But a few years ago, a study conducted by the Center for Science in the Public Interest (CSPI) painted a picture of movie popcorn that's more frightening than the latest version of *Dawn of the Dead.*

The CSPI study found that a large tub of butter-flavored popcorn popped in coconut oil, which is 86 percent saturated fat, contains over 1,600 calories and nearly 130 grams of fat. That's as much fat as in eight Big Macs! Even a small bag (about 5 cups) of butter-flavored popcorn popped in coconut oil packs about 20 grams of fat total, 14 of them saturated.

Most likely, the "butter" is partially hydrogenated soybean oil, which is full of saturated fat and trans fat, an unsaturated fat that raises cholesterol. What's worse, trans fats may cause smaller LDL particles to form, which are more likely to lead to heart disease.

Why do most theaters use coconut oil? People seem to prefer it, says Martin Yadrick, RD, a dietitian in Manhattan Beach, California, and a spokesperson for the American Dietetic Association. Also, coconut oil has a longer shelf life than unsaturated fats such as canola and corn oils, which may make coconut oil a more attractive choice to theater owners.

To avoid movie popcorn's sat-fat attack, consider taking your own air-popped corn to the theater. You might also suggest that the theater offer air-popped corn as well as the oil-popped kind. You never know.

Other options? "Try sprinkling popcorn with Butter Buds, oregano, basil, or sage," suggests Janet Lepke-Harris, RD, a dietitian in Charlotte, North Carolina, and a spokesperson for the American Dietetic Association.

• If you buy microwaveable or ready-to-eat popcorn, opt for "light" varieties; they contain less fat and sodium. Light popcorn isn't necessarily low-fat, however, so check the label for grams of fat and the percentage of calories from fat.

Take note of the serving size, too. Serving sizes for popcorn range from 1 to 3 cups, and that bag of microwave popcorn might contain up to 9 cups. So eating the whole bag would definitely be overdoing it.

• If you must pop your popcorn in oil, opt for canola oil. But make no mistake: Even popcorn popped in canola oil contains fat, notes Martin Yadrick, RD, a dietitian in Manhattan Beach, California, and a spokesperson for the American Dietetic Association. "You'll consume less saturated fat if you use canola oil, but you'll still consume fat," says Yadrick. "So the trick is to use less oil when you make popcorn—or, even better, to air-pop."

Psyllium

More Than Just a Laxative

Psyllium may sound like a vaguely creepy, scientific term. But in reality it's just a natural grain with a husk that's used in many common over-the-counter laxatives, Metamucil being the most recognizable of them.

Psyllium's success at "clearing the plumbing" when needed is historic and well documented. But research has shown that the husks may play an important role in our heart health as well by lowering cholesterol. In fact, the evidence is strong enough that in 1998, the FDA approved a claim that 3 to 12 grams of psyllium taken daily may reduce the risk of heart disease when combined with a diet lower in saturated fat and cholesterol.

Psyllium may be unfamiliar to many people, but the way it helps cholesterol levels is not. Like many cholesterol-lowering foods, it's rich in soluble fiber, a gummy substance that gloms onto cholesterol and flushes it out of the body.

Psyllium is available in supplement form—as powders, wafers, and capsules—and in some breakfast cereals as well. And now, you may have reason to take it for more than just its laxative properties. Here's what the research has shown about psyllium.

Psyllium Solutions

How does psyllium work? Some studies suggest that like other forms of soluble fiber, psyllium prevents the body from reabsorbing a digestive secretion called bile. If the small intestine contains soluble fiber, bile—which contains cholesterol—gets trapped in this gummy stuff and is excreted from the body. Without soluble fiber, the body reabsorbs bile and recycles the cholesterol it contains.

So many studies have been done on psyllium and its effects on cholesterol levels that in 2000, James W. Anderson, MD, professor of medicine and clinical nutrition at the University of Kentucky College of Medicine in Lexington and author of *Dr. Anderson's High-Fiber Fitness Plan,* and his colleagues reviewed the results of eight separate studies for the *American Journal of Clinical Nutrition*. Their meta-analysis included a total of 384 subjects, 272 of whom received some form of psyllium.

After they looked at all the results, the evidence was pretty overwhelming that psyllium plays a role in lowering cholesterol. Dr. Anderson concluded that taking 10.2 grams of psyllium a day along with following a low-fat diet resulted in a 4 percent drop in total cholesterol and a 7 percent drop in "bad" LDL cholesterol while at the same time maintaining triglyceride and "good" HDL levels. The analysis also concluded that psyllium is also well tolerated and safe for most people to take.

The Cereal Ingredient That Surprises Some

As mentioned, you can take psyllium as a powder mixed with water or juice, in capsule or wafer form, or in a psyllium-containing breakfast cereal such as Bran Buds or FiberWise. "Bran Buds are a good choice," says Dr. Anderson. "They contain wheat bran, an insoluble fiber that promotes regularity and health of the colon, as well as soluble fiber, which lowers cholesterol."

If you choose to try a psyllium supplement, follow the recommended dosage on the label, advises Dr. Anderson. Also, for maximum effect, take psyllium with meals. In a study at the University of Toronto, people with mildly high cholesterol who ate Bran Buds for 2 weeks (⅓ cup at breakfast and ⅓ cup at dinner) saw their cholesterol drop by 8 percent. But people who took psyllium powder, mixed with water, between meals had only a minor drop in cholesterol.

Note: There are some instances in which you should not consume this fiber. Don't use psyllium if you're taking certain prescription drugs. Too much psyllium can slow the absorption of heart medication and blood pressure medication, says Dr. Anderson.

Also, if you've had an allergic reaction to laxatives—or if you have any kind of allergy at all—consult your doctor before taking psyllium. This fiber has caused anaphylaxis (a severe allergic reaction) in some people. Such a reaction is rare, however.

Red Wine

Why Redder Is Better

Flaky, crusty, and carb-loaded white bread with every meal. Fatty, creamy, and delicious cheese for dessert. Butter-soaked croissants for breakfast, lunch, and sometimes in between. And less than half the rate of heart attack of Americans.

Which of these four things doesn't belong? Actually, it's a trick question—they *all* belong. That's because they all apply to the French, who for centuries have been eating delicious, rich foods while at the same time having a lower incidence of heart disease and heart attacks than we do here in America. They even have a name for this strange phenomenon—the French paradox. And though theories abound about why the French seem to laugh in the face of a heart-healthy lifestyle, yet still come out on top, the one with the most legs is the idea that the heart protection comes from the extra red wine that the French consume.

An "A" for Alcohol?

Part of the reason that wine is heart healthy is because it contains alcohol. So many studies have confirmed this that it's generally recognized now that moderate drinking can raise levels of "good" HDL cholesterol, prevent the formation of blood clots, lower blood pressure, and prevent damage to the arteries. "The cardiovascular benefits of alcoholic beverages are related to the alcohol itself," says Ann G. Kulze, MD, founder and CEO of Just Wellness, a wellness consulting firm in Mt. Pleasant, South Carolina, and the author of *Dr. Ann's 10-Step Diet.* "Over 100 studies support moderate alcohol consumption's ability to decrease cardiovascular risk."

However, the inherent risks of drinking have always made doctors nervous. That's why the endorsement of drinking is done cautiously and with a strict limit, if it's done at all. The current acceptable limit for "healthy" drinking is two drinks a day if you're a man under 65, and one drink a day if you're a man over 65 or a woman. "As a rule, I don't recommend drinking at all," says Neal Barnard, MD, president of the Physicians Committee for Responsible Medicine in Washington, D.C. "The risks of drinking—such as liver disease, cancer, depression, and alcoholism—are not worth the small amount of benefit that can come from it." For these reasons, the majority of the experts we spoke with stuck by a simple, straightforward mantra—if you don't drink, don't start.

What Else Is in Wine?

Okay, now that we're clear on the possible benefits—and great risks—associated with alcohol, suppose you were to drink moderately on occasion. And suppose you were to drink red wine instead of, say, a glass of Scotch, a can of beer, or even a glass of white wine. The question that researchers have been trying to get at for some time now is this: Would that red wine provide you with more benefit than the other alcoholic choices? In other words, is there more going on in a glass of red wine than in alcohol alone?

Though the studies and expert opinions on this topic are mixed, it appears that as more research is done, it looks more and more like something else is going on inside wine to give it unique heart-healthy properties.

"Red wine is felt to have additional benefits over and above those related to its alcohol content, as a result of the polyphenols, phytochemicals, and other antioxidants it contains," says Dr. Kulze. "Resveratrol is one of a whole laundry list of such agents. Benefits are likely related to the combination of these many different bioactive substances found within wine."

Just to clarify, polyphenols and phytochemicals are two types of flavonoids, chemical compounds found in plants that appear to have strong antioxidant properties. And antioxidants are a huge factor in the fight against heart disease. Though they don't specifically prevent cholesterol from developing, they do prevent it from oxidizing—depositing itself along the arterial walls and causing damage to the arteries.

Resveratrol is just one of these flavonoid compounds found within red wine. And despite its funny name, this fungus-fighting chemical from the skin of grapes has certainly garnered a lot of attention in the press recently.

According to John D. Folts, PhD, director of the University of Wisconsin Coronary Artery Thrombosis Research and Prevention Lab at the University of Wisconsin Hospital and Clinics in Madison and one of the leading researchers on red wine, however, resveratrol might not even be the most important compound within red wine. "A lot of research has speculated that resveratrol may help lower cholesterol, and one study showed that purified resveratrol appeared to lower cholesterol in rats," he says. "However, there is only a small amount of it in red wine or grape juice, and the research showing benefit from resveratrol has required much larger amounts." What's more, adds Dr. Folts, "resveratrol didn't show platelet-inhibiting properties in our studies."

So does this mean that red wine's heart-healthy antioxidant compounds aren't quite all they're cracked up to be? Quite the contrary, says Dr. Folts. Instead, he believes that it's a combination of the compounds found in the grape seeds and skins to offer benefits. This is yet another reason that it's best to focus on the whole foods, rather than trying to pick out the individual components that can help.

Does the Type of Wine Matter?

Thus far, the evidence has been pretty clear that the grapes—and the compounds within them—may give wine an edge over its heart-healthy alcoholic competitors. But white wine has grapes in it, too. So why does red wine get all the attention?

As it turns out, there's a simple reason for this—and it has to do with how red wine is made. "Red wine differs from white wine or other alcoholic beverages because in red wine the skins of the grapes are in contact with the juice of the wine for a long period of time, allowing many of the important plant chemicals (the flavonoids) to enter into the wine," says Ralph Felder, MD, PhD, section chief for cardiovascular nutrition at the Good Samaritan Medical Center in Phoenix and author of *The Bonus Years Diet*. "The flavonoids have antioxidant properties that potentially are very important in maintaining the Teflon-like lining of the blood vessels, helping to dilate the blood vessels, and preventing clots from forming."

The science certainly seems to back up Dr. Felder's notion that red wine has more antioxidants than white wine. In 2006, researchers attempted to measure the antioxidant potential of more than 1,000 common foods. Not

Heart-Healthy Indulgences

Fish and Wine: The Perfect Heart-Healthy Meal

The heart-healthy properties of fish, particularly fish rich in omega-3 fatty acids, have been well documented in recent years. Now it seems that those benefits can become even greater when you pair a glass of red wine or two with the meal.

In a Danish study, 291 men and women who were suspected of having ischemic heart disease, a condition in which there is inadequate blood flow to the heart, were surveyed about how much fish and wine they consumed. The researchers then measured the levels of omega-3 fatty acids in their blood fats.

As it turned out, the people with higher levels of omega-3s had higher heart rate variability (HRV) than those with low levels. Simply put, low HRV is a significant indicator of sudden cardiac death in people with ischemic heart disease. The results seemed pretty conclusive that eating fish decreased the risk of an unexpected fatal heart attack. (Oily fish like salmon, tuna, and mackerel have more generous amounts of omega-3s than pale, lean fish like haddock or flounder.)

What's more, the researchers noted that people who ate a lot of fish often tended to drink more wine. While wine may have some positive health effects of its own, it seems that consuming wine and fish together can maximize your health benefits.

surprisingly, red wine was in the top 15, while white wine wasn't even close to being as rich in antioxidants.

As it turns out, it may be more than just the color of the wine that determines its antioxidant potential. "A recent study found that red wines from Sardinia and Southwest France have the highest concentrations of the most efficacious red wine antioxidants," says Dr. Kulze. Suddenly, this whole "French paradox" thing is beginning to make a lot more sense.

Heart Protection in a Glass

Though what looks good in theory doesn't always pan out when put under the microscope, the good news about red wine is that the studies look as promising as the ideas behind them. Here's what researchers have found.

One French study took the alcohol-versus-wine challenge head-on by pitting them against one another in a group of 56 healthy young men. Over 14 days, the men drank about an ounce a day of one of three beverages: red wine, a different alcoholic beverage, or alcohol-free red wine. Though both sources of alcohol increased levels of "good" HDL cholesterol, the alcoholic beverage increased triglycerides, while the wine did not. There was no effect from the alcohol-free red wine other than decreasing HDL. The researchers concluded that red wine seemed to have a slight edge over other forms of alcohol.

Another study indicated that drinking wine or other alcoholic beverages might prevent blood clotting by boosting levels of tissue-type plasminogen activator, or tPA. In a study of more than 600 men, those who reported consuming two or more drinks a day had 35 percent more tPA in their blood than men who said they rarely or never drank.

When it comes to heart attack prevention, however, red wine seems to be on an even keel with other forms of alcohol. In a study at Harvard University and Brigham and Women's Hospital in Boston, researchers examined the relationship between heart attack and the type of alcoholic beverages consumed. Their analysis showed that moderate drinkers had a lower risk of heart attack than nondrinkers, thanks to the boost provided in HDL levels. But they could not distinguish whether one type of alcohol provided any greater benefit than another.

Though the differences between red wine and other forms of alcohol seemed rather ambiguous in this particular study, other research has shown that the antioxidants in red wine clearly play a role that's distinct from that of wine's alcohol content. One example of this was at the University of California, Davis, where researchers collected blood samples from people with normal cholesterol levels. They then removed the LDL cholesterol from those samples and mixed this LDL with phenolic (antioxidant) compounds that they collected from red wine. The results were pretty dramatic: The phenolic compounds reduced the oxidation of LDL cholesterol by 60 to 98 percent. Oxidation is a chemical process that makes LDL more harmful and more likely to enter the arterial walls and accelerate hardening of the arteries, coronary thrombosis, and stroke.

A separate study at Queen Elizabeth Hospital in Birmingham, England, provided more direct evidence that red wine seems to increase antioxidant activity in the blood. Researchers had 10 people consume two lunches over the course of 2 days. At one of the lunches, each person drank a glass of red wine. At the other, they drank no wine at all. A half-hour after each meal, each volunteer gave the first of several blood samples taken over a 4-hour period.

After the wine meal, the antioxidant levels in the people's blood rose, reaching a peak after 90 minutes. More significantly, their antioxidant levels were higher than those required to inhibit the oxidation of LDL cholesterol in test-tube experiments. After the wine-free meal, the blood showed little change in antioxidant activity.

See also Alcohol, Flavonoids, Grape Juice, Grape Seed Extract

Smoking Cessation
Yet Another Reason to Quit

If you still smoke, chances are good that your eyes gloss over when you hear yet another reason you should put down the pack. But let's face it—with mounting research to show that smoking has a dramatic impact on heart health—another reminder is always prudent.

The evidence is so overwhelming that smoking is one of the American Heart Association's "big six"—the six risk factors for heart disease that you can do something about, along with such heavy hitters as high blood cholesterol, high blood pressure, inactivity, obesity, and diabetes. When you consider that smokers have two to four times the risk of developing heart disease and twice the risk of dying from a heart attack as nonsmokers, it's easy to see why smoking made the list. In fact, even exposure to secondhand smoke has been shown to increase the risk of heart disease in nonsmokers.

When it comes to cholesterol levels and smoking, the news is just as bad. A number of studies have shown that smokers have less "good" HDL cholesterol, more "bad" LDL cholesterol, and higher total cholesterol. And for some reason, smokers with elevated cholesterol are more likely to develop heart disease than nonsmokers with elevated cholesterol. Let's explore the research to find out exactly why this is.

Studies against Smoking

It's not hard to find studies that look at the connection between smoking and cholesterol. One of the largest that isolated smoking as a risk factor was a Chinese study that compared 6,097 smokers to 841 nonsmokers. Across the board, the smokers had lower HDL levels and higher LDL levels. In addition, the more the people in the study smoked, the worse their ratio of HDL to LDL became.

Literally hundreds of studies have come to the same conclusion. But what was somewhat perplexing is why smokers are more likely to get heart disease than nonsmokers with similar cholesterol levels. As it turns out, the reason for this is simple: Just as in the lungs, smoking literally robs the arteries of oxygen. This hastens the damage and hardening of the arteries (arteriosclerosis), which in turn makes it more likely that cholesterol will be deposited on the vessel walls (atherosclerosis), leading to heart disease. This deadly one-two punch of higher cholesterol and damaged arteries goes a long way toward explaining why smokers' risks of heart disease and heart attack are so great.

The Road to Recovery

Luckily, the news isn't all bad when it comes to smoking and your heart. After all, the incentive to quit is rising by the day. Every year, about 1.3 million Americans stop smoking. Though about 48 million Americans—about 23 percent of the population—still smoke, that number is down from 42 percent in 1965. Since that year, 40 percent of people who smoked at one time have kicked the habit.

And when you do quit, your heart will thank you faster than you might think. After just a year, your risk of developing heart disease drops by half. After 15 years, your risk of heart disease is the same as if you had never smoked at all.

Getting Ready to Stop

Quitting smoking isn't easy. But you can make it easier. In one study, researchers from the Arizona Program for Nicotine and Tobacco Research at the University of Arizona in Tucson found that almost two times as many smokers who used bupropion, a prescription antidepressant approved as a smoking-cessation aid and sold under the brand name Zyban, were able to abstain from tobacco as those who used either nicotine patches or a placebo (inactive substance). (A nicotine patch delivers enough nicotine through the skin to reduce withdrawal symptoms and help wean you off inhaled smoke that damages your heart and lungs.) The following tips can also help.

• Keep a smoking journal for 2 weeks before you quit, suggest C. Richard Conti, MD, and Diana Tonnessen in their book *Beating the Odds against Heart Disease and High Cholesterol.* Jot down the circumstances that most often prompt you to light up: during your coffee break, after dinner, while chatting on the phone, when you're feeling lonely or bored, and so forth.

• After a week, review your journal, pinpointing circumstances that prompt you to smoke. Then list alternatives to smoking during those times. If your journal shows that you tend to smoke after meals, for example, brush your teeth or take a walk instead.

• Decide whether you want to quit smoking all at once—that is, "cold turkey"—or taper off. While you may decide to stop smoking gradually, there's evidence that most successful quitters go cold turkey.

• Pick a Quit Day and mark it on your calendar. Make it no later than 1 week away. Many experts suggest quitting on a weekend, when most people have better control of their time, surroundings, and circumstances.

• Get a buddy to help you make it through the quitting process. This person can be a nonsmoker, a former smoker, or a smoker who will quit with you. Call your buddy when the going gets rough.

• Tell your family, friends, and co-workers about your Quit Day. Letting people know about your decision to quit smoking will help hold you to your resolve.

• Call or write your local chapter of the American Heart Association, the American Cancer Society, or the American Lung Association and ask for their free brochures and pamphlets on smoking cessation.

• Get some kind of exercise. "Women who work out are conscious of their health and tend not to smoke," says Myra Muramoto, MD, associate professor of Family and Community Medicine and director of the University of Arizona Physicians Healthcare Quit and Win Tobacco Cessation Program.

A Quit-Day Checklist

Here's what to do when Quit Day dawns.

• Throw away all of your cigarettes and matches. Soak the cigarettes in water so you can't scrounge them out of the trash.

• Hide all the ashtrays. Better yet, get rid of them.

• Lay in a supply of healthy snacks such as celery, carrots, apples, sunflower seeds, and air-popped popcorn. They'll keep your mouth and fingers busy without wreaking havoc on your shape.

• Take a long walk or visit a nonsmoking environment such as a library, museum, or movie theater.

Patching Up HDL

Sure, quitting smoking can increase "good" HDL cholesterol. But if you're using nicotine transdermal replacement (better known as the nicotine patch) to kick the habit, you may be wondering if the patch will continue to lower HDL levels. Maybe not, according to one study.

Researchers at the University of Minnesota Medical School in Minneapolis examined the effect of the nicotine patch on people who abstained from smoking. After 6 weeks, these folks' blood pressure, heart rates, and "bad" LDL cholesterol dropped while their HDL cholesterol and triglycerides increased—even while they were using active nicotine patches.

If you're considering using the patch, talk with your doctor first about how it can become part of a comprehensive smoking-cessation program.

• Plan to have your teeth cleaned to get rid of tobacco stains. Resolve to keep them that way.

• Avoid stressful situations and smoking environments (bars, for example). Spend as much time as possible in places where smoking isn't permitted.

What about withdrawal symptoms? Well, there's good news and bad news. The bad news first: About 80 percent of smokers experience such symptoms when they quit, from headaches and fatigue to nausea, diarrhea, and constipation. Some people also feel anxious, depressed, or irritable or have trouble sleeping. The good news: Withdrawal symptoms tend to subside in 2 to 3 days, after the nicotine has left your body, and will be gone—or nearly so—within a couple of weeks.

Staying Off 'Em

Most people are capable of quitting smoking. The key is to not start again. Here are three ways to kick the habit for good.

• Be alert for "smoke signals." One study identified the four most likely relapse scenarios: during social drinking, after a meal, while feeling anxious at work, and while feeling depressed or anxious when at home alone.

• Learn a relaxation technique, such as deep breathing or progressive relaxation. If smoking helps you relax, "you're likely to feel more stressed when you quit smoking unless you have other ways to manage stress that aren't centered on cigarettes," says Dean Ornish, MD, president and director of the Preventive Medicine Research Institute in Sausalito, California, and author of *Dr. Dean Ornish's Program for Reversing Heart Disease*.

• On an index card, list two or three of your most important reasons for quitting smoking. Stash the card in your pocket or purse, where you used to keep your cigarettes. Pull it out and go over the list often, particularly when you feel the urge to smoke.

See also Exercise, Stress Management, Walking

Soy Foods
The Plant That Can Take Meat's Place

In years past, soy foods were strictly the domain of "health nuts." More often than not, they were embraced by vegetarians, who needed a suitable replacement for the protein normally provided by meat in a diet. Take a stroll through the supermarket today, though, and it's clear to see that this "fringe" food has gone mainstream. Everything from hot dogs and hamburgers to milk and ice cream now has a soy-based substitute.

These foods are for more than just vegetarians, too. There are a lot of good reasons to add soy to a healthy diet, particularly as a substitute for meat products. And though you may have heard some bad news about soy over the past few years, we'll explain why it's still a great choice for your heart.

Soy's Up-and-Down Road

If you've followed the news about soy over the last decade, chances are you've been on quite a roller-coaster ride. In the late 1990s, soy was almost unanimously hailed as the next great cholesterol savior. In 1999, the FDA labeled foods that contained a certain amount of soy protein as heart protective, and in 2000, the American Heart Association followed suit by giving its own endorsement to foods with soy protein.

Then the backlash began. In 2006, the American Heart Association reviewed the results of 22 studies of the effects of soy protein on cholesterol levels. While levels of "bad" LDL cholesterol decreased in all of the studies, the results were only statistically significant in eight of the studies. The soy protein also had little effect on triglycerides and "good" HDL cholesterol in most of the studies.

Moreover, most of the positive benefits came from consuming soy protein at a level of 50 grams a day or more, which is half of the recommended daily intake of protein, and an unrealistic amount for most people to consume. As a result of these findings, the American Heart Association now recommends against taking soy or isoflavone supplements to reduce the risk of heart disease.

However, most experts, including those who conducted the review for the American Heart Association, are quick to point out that these findings by no means slam the door on soy. "The backlash on soy has been almost as overblown as the initial findings on soy protein," says Christopher Gardner, PhD, of the Stanford Prevention Research Center at Stanford University Medical Center. "The bottom line is that soy is a very healthy food choice."

Ann G. Kulze, MD, founder and CEO of Just Wellness, a wellness consulting firm in Mt. Pleasant, South Carolina, and the author of *Dr. Ann's 10-Step Diet*, agrees, adding that the most benefit can be obtained from soy by replacing meat and animal products in your diet with soy products. "It's particularly beneficial to work toward substituting soy foods, like soy burgers, for red meat that is high in saturated fats and often contains hormonal residues along with other harmful chemicals," she says. "This way, you get the nutritional benefits of soy while simultaneously displacing unhealthy fat calories from your diet."

Recently, Dr. Gardner conducted a study that helped show exactly that. He and his colleagues placed 120 adults with high cholesterol on a low-fat diet. Sixty-one of them were on a diet of common "low-fat" products, such as skinless chicken breasts, potatoes, and low-fat cheeses and dressings. The other 59 replaced the fatty elements of their diet with healthier foods such as soy foods, vegetables, beans, and nuts.

After 4 weeks, both groups experienced improvements in total and LDL cholesterol. But the group eating soy and other healthy food choices saw their levels drop almost twice as much as the other group: 18-point declines in total cholesterol and 14-point declines in LDL cholesterol.

The Science of Soy

How does soy help our hearts? According to Dr. Kulze, there are three reasons: "Soy has three superstar ingredients for decreasing cholesterol," she says. "Soluble fiber, soy protein, and plant sterols."

Soluble fiber's role in reducing cholesterol is well documented. This fiber literally grabs onto cholesterol and ushers it out of the body. And the role of plant sterols in reducing cholesterol is outlined in detail on page 135. What's unique about soy, however, is that its protein also seems to play a role. But as the American Heart Association's 2006 review has shown, this role is somewhat controversial.

One theory is that the protein in soy helps because of the protein it replaces in the diet. By eating a plant-based protein rather than a meat-based protein, you get the benefits without all the harmful saturated fat. And though soy is moderately high in fat, it's still a better choice than a slab of steak.

You Don't Have to Eat Tofu (Unless You Want To)

With all this great news about the benefits of soy, you'd think more people would be eating it by now. The problem may be the misleading perception that there is one choice for soy food and only one—tofu.

Tofu is undoubtedly the most well-known soy food. Like pasta, this soft, mild-tasting substance takes on the flavor of whatever it's cooked with, so it tastes equally good in the spiciest chili and the creamiest cheesecake—and in virtually any other dish.

How to Speak Soy

Don't know tofu from tempeh? Relax—this primer can help introduce you to the joy of soy.

Isolated soy protein. A powdered form of soy protein found in powdered weight-loss drinks and other products.

Meat analogs. These soy-based "meats" include cold cuts, bacon, sausage, franks, and burgers.

Soy flour. Made by flaking and grinding roasted soybeans. You can replace up to 20 percent of regular flour with soy flour. Also, use defatted soy flour; the regular variety is very high in fat.

Soy milk. A creamy, milklike drink made from ground soaked soybeans and water. You can drink soy milk straight, pour it over cereal, or substitute it for whole or fat-free milk in other dishes.

Tempeh. Cakes of cooked, fermented soybeans, laced with a mold that gives tempeh its distinctive flavor. Tempeh is usually grilled, roasted, steamed, or added to soups.

Texturized soy protein. Made from soy flour, TSP is a meat substitute that is used to replace part or all of the meat in chili or hamburgers. You buy TSP in dry form and add water before use.

Tofu. A creamy white, soft cake made from curded soy milk. Tofu can be sliced, diced, or crumbled and used in soups, stir-fries, casseroles, and sandwiches.

But if tofu isn't to your liking, you can still enjoy your soy. Today, most supermarkets carry a wide variety of soy beverages, canned or frozen soybeans, soy nuts, and commercially prepared soy-based products, from cheese and yogurt to meat analogs (meat substitutes made from soy protein).

Dr. Kulze recommends getting a very reasonable amount of soy foods daily: two servings. "This can be as simple as having soy milk on your cereal or in a smoothie for breakfast, and a handful of soy nuts as a midafternoon snack," she says.

Keep in mind, though, that wolfing down tofu or soy-based breakfast "sausage" on top of a burgers-and-fries diet isn't likely to reduce your cholesterol. It works only as part of a low-fat, low-cholesterol diet. And according to experts, replacing a portion of the meat and dairy foods in your diet with their tasty soy counterparts can be a heart-smart move.

You'll Never Miss the Meat

Look for soy-based products, from tofu (often found in the produce section) to commercially prepared "meat products" such as vegetable burgers, in your local supermarket. You'll probably find isolated soy protein (ISP), texturized soy protein (TSP), and tempeh in health food stores. The following tips can help you enjoy your soy.

- Mix mashed tofu with diced vegetables, herbs, and spices and use it as a vegetable dip or sandwich filling.
- Add cubed tofu to stir-fried vegetables.
- Crumble tofu into spaghetti sauce or chili.

A Beginner's Guide to Tofu
Want to give tofu a try? Follow these tips.

- Select low-fat or fat-free tofu. Regular versions can get anywhere from 30 to over 50 percent of their calories from fat.
- Select tofu curded with calcium sulfate. This variety contains 860 milligrams of calcium, compared with 258 milligrams of calcium in tofu curded with nigari (magnesium chloride).
- Buy tofu in sealed packages. Tofu that sits in water and is exposed to the open air has been found to contain high levels of bacteria.

- Pour soy milk over cereal or substitute it for whole milk in soups, cakes, puddings, and other dishes that call for milk.
- Combine chilled vanilla soy milk and chilled coffee in a frosted mug for a refreshing "iced soy cappuccino."
- Grill sliced tempeh, then top it with regular burger fixings.
- Add ISP to baked goods.

See also Fiber, Plant Stanols and Sterols

Stress Management
Relax . . . Your Heart Will Thank You

Diet may be the biggest concern when it comes to cholesterol and overall heart health. But among the other lifestyle factors that play a role, stress levels are certainly a concern as well.

Though health experts almost unanimously agree that controlling stress is a good idea, what's interesting is that a link between stress and heart disease hasn't been definitively proven. Part of the reason for this is that stress, while very real, is an incredibly difficult thing to measure in a scientific study. Also, it's unclear whether it's stress alone that contributes to heart disease or whether stress encourages other risk factors such as eating poorly, smoking, and not exercising.

Regardless of what the true connection is, controlling stress has been shown to help the heart, particularly in preventing a second heart attack. And in cases of heart failure, keeping stress under wraps is absolutely vital to your survival. Read on to explore the role of stress in heart disease and learn some ways to keep it under control.

The Stone Age Response

Ironically, the same physiological reaction to stress that helped our caveman ancestors outrun predators may play some role in modern man's (and woman's) proclivity for developing coronary heart disease. This reaction, called the fight-or-flight response, is your inborn red-alert system that readies your body to repel a threat—real or imagined.

During the fight-or-flight response, your body releases stress hormones such as cortisol and adrenaline into your bloodstream. These hormones speed up your breathing, increase your heart rate, and accelerate the flow of blood to your arms and legs (the better to help you flee). But if your body triggers this inner alarm dozens of times a day, it can lay the foundation for heart disease.

"Stress seems to accelerate the depositing of plaque into the arteries independent of its effect on blood cholesterol," says Dean Ornish, MD, president and director of the Preventive Medicine Research Institute in Sausalito, California. In other words, he says, the harmful part of stress has less to do with its effect on cholesterol than its effect on the arteries themselves.

"Stress can make your arteries constrict, which can reduce blood flow to the heart," says Dr. Ornish. "It can cause something called plaque hemorrhage, which is a rupture of the lining of the arteries that can lead to the arteries becoming obstructed. And stress can cause blood to clot faster, which can lead to a heart attack."

Arterial Enemies: Beef, Butter, and . . . Burnout?

Think burgers and butter are your arteries' only enemies? Think again. Years ago, a well-known study demonstrated that accountants' blood cholesterol skyrocketed by as many as 100 points above their usual levels during tax season. Another study showed that students' blood cholesterol spiked during exams. Here are a few other studies linking stress with stratospheric cholesterol counts.

Researchers at the University of Pittsburgh had 44 healthy men and women either take a complicated computerized test to raise their stress levels or rest quietly for 20 minutes. Blood samples were taken before and after the test and the rest period. Those who took the test showed significant increases in total and "bad" LDL cholesterol.

Researchers in Israel tracked 104 men between the ages of 24 and 68. These men didn't have cardiovascular disease, but they did have highly stressful jobs and were defined by the researchers as "burned out." (The study defined burnout as a mix of physical fatigue, mental exhaustion, and other factors.)

After controlling for age, weight, and other factors, the researchers discovered that the total cholesterol of the most burned-out men was 14 percent higher than that of the most relaxed men. What's more, the most stressed-out men had significantly higher LDL cholesterol, the kind that wreaks the most cardiovascular damage.

Researchers at the Brown University Medical School in Providence, Rhode Island, drew blood from 114 men and women, then administered two psychological tests used to measure anxiety and responses to it. After factoring in age, weight, and smoking habits, the researchers found that men who repressed their feelings tended to have higher cholesterol than men who didn't. Interestingly, women who repressed negative emotions had lower total and LDL cholesterol than women who didn't. One researcher has suggested that emotional stress may exert a lower physiological toll on women than on men.

Learning to Let Go

The bad news: There's no way to avoid stress. The good news: You can learn to cope with stress in a more heart-healthy manner. So before you come apart at the seams, consider your cholesterol level and try these stress-busting tips.

• Breathe deeply. "Your breathing is a reflection of your mental state. It's a bridge between your mind and your body, and it can be used to change your frame of mind," says Dr. Ornish. "If you're feeling anxious, your breathing becomes more rapid and shallow. But consciously making yourself breathe more slowly and deeply can help calm you."

• Get some real exercise. According to experts, aerobic exercise, such as a brisk stroll, can help reduce the amount of stress-producing hormones barreling through your bloodstream. "Exercise is a great stress-reducing tool," says Peter O. Kwiterovich Jr., MD, professor of medicine and director of the Lipid Research and Atherosclerosis Unit at Johns Hopkins University School of Medicine in Baltimore and author of *The Johns Hopkins Complete Guide for Preventing and Reversing Heart Disease*. "I recommend regular aerobic exercise. Try to exercise a half hour a day, three or four times a week."

• Don't spread yourself too thin—it's a major cause of stress, says James W. Anderson, MD, professor of medicine and clinical nutrition at the University of Kentucky College of Medicine in Lexington and author of *Dr.*

Anderson's High-Fiber Fitness Plan. "Schedule your time carefully and learn to say no when you need to," he advises.

• Take 10. When you need it, give yourself 10 minutes to relax and focus on yourself.

Yoga: The New-Age Cholesterol Buster

If you've ever been interested in giving yoga a try, here's another reason: Yoga has been shown in studies to be a proven stress buster and relaxation technique. Some studies indicate that yoga can slow the heart rate, relax breathing, and even lower blood pressure in some people.

While it's unclear whether yoga can directly lower cholesterol, yoga's success as a stress buster makes it a great addition to any heart-healthy regimen. One small study in India even showed that yoga directly lowered cholesterol and triglycerides in six healthy young men.

If you're interested in trying yoga yourself, make sure you find a class that focuses on relaxation rather than pushing the body to new limits, which some advanced classes try to do. The key is to do your research up front and be clear with the instructor when you discuss what you're looking for in a yoga class. Then, see if you can sit in on a class or two to make sure it's a good fit for you.

In the meantime, here is a stretching technique you can try at home to relieve stress.

1. While standing or sitting, place your arms behind your back and clasp your hands. If your hands don't meet comfortably, "cheat" by holding the ends of a towel.

2. Stretch upward and outward. Feel the stretch across your chest (but don't stretch so far that it hurts).

3. Take a deep breath. As you exhale, continue to stretch, opening up your chest and keeping your hands clasped.

4. Continue to take full, deep breaths, drawing air down into your belly and letting it out again. After several minutes, take one more breath and slowly unclasp your hands.

In addition, here's a simple breathing exercise that can help you relax.

1. Sit comfortably in a chair or on a couch. Keep your spine fairly straight and your shoulders back and relaxed.

2. With your eyes closed, close off your right nostril with your right thumb and take 26 long, deep breaths through your left nostril. Then close off your left nostril with your left thumb and repeat the process, breathing through your right nostril. Let yourself become completely calm and try to enter a peaceful, focused state.

• Think before you snack. Before you begin stuffing your face, ask yourself: Am I really hungry or just stressed? To fight the urge, wait a few minutes, go for a walk, eat a piece of fruit first, or if it's late at night, just try to go to bed.

• Pamper yourself. Take time for a relaxing massage, a long walk, or whatever makes you happy.

• Don't forget your friends. Making regular time for your friends and family is a great way to bust stress.

• Always laugh. Finding humor in everyday life is the best way to keep things in perspective.

See also Exercise, Walking

Triglyceride Control
Cholesterol's Lesser-Known Cousin

When it comes to risk factors for heart disease, your blood cholesterol level is one number you definitely want to be familiar with. But it's by no means the only number you need to know.

Another blood fat, while lesser known, can play a role in heart disease and atherosclerosis. This type of blood fat is known as triglycerides.

Both triglycerides and cholesterol circulate in the bloodstream with the help of lipoproteins. But while the body uses cholesterol to build cells and

What's Your Level?

Like cholesterol, triglycerides are measured in milligrams/deciliter. Here are the National Cholesterol Education Program's guidelines for triglyceride levels.

Less than 150—Normal
150 to 199—Borderline high
200 to 499—High
500 and above—Very high

hormones, it stores triglycerides for extra energy. After you eat, any calories that your body doesn't need are converted into triglycerides. Overeat frequently, and you could develop high triglycerides, which present risks to the arteries and heart similar to those of high cholesterol.

In fact, the risks of triglycerides are great enough that the federal government has lowered the bar on how many triglycerides are considered "borderline high," "high," and "very high," making these guidelines more stringent than ever before. (For more information on triglyceride levels, see "What's Your Level?") In addition, the government has put greater emphasis on screening for triglycerides and has urged doctors to tell their patients with high triglycerides about the importance of losing weight and exercising.

The Trouble with Triglycerides

While the exact way in which triglycerides contribute to heart disease isn't entirely clear, they are certainly a risk factor, as high triglycerides are commonly present at the same time as other risk factors such as high total cholesterol, high LDL cholesterol, and low HDL cholesterol. What's more, people with diabetes tend to have high levels of triglycerides, making it even more critical for them to keep an eye on this complicating factor.

Doctors have a number of theories about how triglycerides might contribute more directly to heart disease. One idea is that triglycerides in the body get "remetabolized" in the liver and converted into artery-damaging LDL cholesterol. What's more, the LDL particles formed by triglyceride

---

Drop "Tri's" with Omega-3s

The omega-3 fatty acids found in fish like salmon, mackerel, and tuna, as well as in fish oil supplements, have shown a lot of benefits when it comes to heart health. And one area where omega-3s may have big-time promise is in lowering triglyceride levels.

In one study at the Oregon Health and Science University in Portland, people with very high triglycerides (over 1,000 milligrams/deciliter, or mg/dl) saw their levels drop below 500 mg/dl with the addition of 3 to 4 grams of fish oil a day.

This high dose of fish oil can only be obtained from a fish oil supplement, so you'll want to speak with your doctor before beginning a fish oil supplement regimen. In addition, benefit can also be obtained from eating two servings of fish every week.

metabolism are small and dense, which may be even more harmful to the arteries.

Other studies have found that high triglycerides can cause a number of other problems. One study showed that high triglycerides, when paired up with low levels of "good" HDL cholesterol, presented an increased risk of death from heart disease. This is a particularly scary scenario, as people with high triglycerides and low HDL can often present normal total cholesterol readings.

When researchers in Norway analyzed the triglyceride levels in 24,535 middle-aged women, they found that as triglyceride readings increased, so did deaths related to coronary heart disease, as well as deaths from all causes.

Heart-Healthy Indulgences

Peanut Butter: It's Not Just for Kids

Once a staple in children's lunchboxes and often a grown-up favorite as well, peanut butter fell a bit out of favor a while ago when it was indicted as being too high in calories.

Surprise! Studies have now shown that peanut butter can aid in weight loss and cholesterol reduction. Peanut butter is rich in monounsaturated fats, which are considered beneficial to heart health. A study by Brigham and Women's Hospital and Harvard Medical School in Boston showed that dieters who ate large amounts of monounsaturated fats lost weight. And, thanks to the chemical structure of monounsaturated fats, peanut butter can help lower levels of triglycerides and LDL cholesterol while maintaining HDL levels.

Other studies suggest additional benefits: sizeable drops in fibrinogen (a blood-clotting protein that's been linked to coronary artery disease when it's too high), glucose, insulin, and small, dense LDL particles. All of these factors can help to prevent a heart attack.

Here are some suggestions for incorporating peanut butter into your grown-up diet.

- Spread a tablespoon on whole grain toast.

- In PB&J sandwiches, substitute fresh, sliced strawberries for jelly or jam.

The researchers found no relationship between triglycerides and mortality in 25,058 men, however.

Researchers at Johns Hopkins University School of Medicine in Baltimore examined the relationship between cardiovascular disease and various blood fat measurements (total, HDL and LDL cholesterol, and triglycerides) in about 1,400 women ages 50 to 69. Over a 14-year period, high triglycerides (over 200 milligrams/deciliter, or mg/dl), particularly in combination with low HDL levels (under 50 mg/dl), were associated with an increased risk of death from heart disease. The researchers concluded that elevated triglycerides are an independent predictor of death from cardiovascular disease in women. Further, they recommended that "cholesterol screening guidelines should be reevaluated to reflect the importance of HDL and triglyceride levels in determining risk in women."

People with high triglyceride levels may have more problems than others in lowering their LDL cholesterol, according to a study conducted at the Alton Ochsner Medical Foundation in New Orleans. Researchers followed the progress of 313 people who were enrolled in a rehabilitation program after having heart trouble. All of them had high cholesterol, and 39 had elevated triglycerides. The group was put on a low-fat, low-cholesterol diet for 3 months.

By the end of the study, the group as a whole had significant improvements in total, LDL, and HDL cholesterol. But the people with high triglyceride levels had no significant improvement in LDL cholesterol or in the ratio of LDL to HDL. According to the researchers, people with high triglycerides may need more aggressive nondrug treatment to improve their cholesterol profiles.

Cutting These Fats Down to Size

Most experts advise taking steps to lower high triglycerides, especially if you have low HDL cholesterol or high LDL cholesterol. "A high triglyceride level is a warning sign in many patients who have a predisposition for coronary heart disease," says Peter O. Kwiterovich Jr., MD, professor of medicine and director of the Lipid Research and Atherosclerosis Unit at Johns Hopkins University School of Medicine in Baltimore and author of *The Johns Hopkins Complete Guide for Preventing and Reversing Heart Disease*. "It needs to be taken care of."

Fortunately, say most doctors, you can usually lower a high triglyceride level with lifestyle changes. Here are some of the most common triglyceride-lowering strategies.

• Lose weight. "Triglycerides respond very well to weight reduction," says Dr. Kwiterovich. "Losing as little as 5 to 10 pounds will significantly lower your triglycerides."

• Avoid alcohol. While studies have shown that a drink or two a day can help raise HDL cholesterol, alcohol can actually raise triglycerides by lowering the concentration of an enzyme used to break them down. "Even having a glass of wine with dinner every night can substantially raise triglycerides in people who are overweight or who have hereditary triglyceride problems," says Thomas Bersot, MD, PhD, clinical professor of medicine at the University of California, San Francisco.

• Avoid refined carbohydrates and sugars. Partially refined carbohydrates, including white flour and white rice; refined sugars such as those in candy; and even some high-sugar fruit juices such as orange juice will raise triglycerides in some people. Instead, choose whole grain sources of carbohydrates that are rich in fiber such as whole wheat bread, brown rice, barley, and rolled oats.

• Exercise. Even walking just 2 miles a day is enough to drop triglycerides and boost HDL cholesterol.

• Consider medication. If all else fails, your doctor may advise medication to help lower very high triglycerides. All drugs have potentially adverse effects, so discuss any possible downsides to the use of medication with your doctor.

Vegetables

The Cornerstone of Heart-Healthy Eating

Have you ever noticed that vegetables usually get second billing to fruits in the English language? Whenever we talk about them, it's "fruits and vegetables"—seldom the other way around.

According to Christopher Gardner, PhD, of the Stanford Prevention Research Center at Stanford University Medical Center, vegetables soon won't be an afterthought anymore. "You might notice on the American Heart Association Web site, as well as other sources, that the language is changing to 'vegetables and fruits,'" he says.

When you think about the research behind this heart-healthy duo of foods, it makes sense that veggies would get top billing, adds Dr. Gardner. They're lower in sugar than many fruits and positively brimming with antioxidants, flavonoids, and other heart-healthy compounds.

Now that's not to say that fruits are a bad food choice. In fact, they're a great choice compared to all the junk food that's out there. But when you consider that vegetables are a *better* choice than fruits—well, that just shows how great vegetables really are for your heart health.

Some facts about veggies and heart health will come as no surprise. They're virtually fat free—meaning they're always a smart, heart-healthy food choice. They're brimming with fiber, so they have the natural stuff that can remove excess cholesterol from the bloodstream. In addition, they're packed with antioxidants, which have been shown in studies to enhance blood flow and reduce the oxidation of "bad" LDL cholesterol in the bloodstream. Oxidation is a chemical process that researchers believe increases the likelihood that LDL will collect in the arteries.

Experts know the benefits of produce, which is why the federal government recently upped the daily recommendations for fruits and veggies from five servings a day to a whopping nine. If some newer research is any indication, we have even more great reasons to chow down on more of them.

Heart-Healthy Indulgences

Real Salad Dressing: Oil Isn't All Bad

If you don't go overboard, dressings made with oil can have real benefits for your body and its engine, the heart.

Dressings made with canola or olive oil supply cholesterol-reducing monounsaturated fats, and those made with canola or walnut oil are good sources of alpha-linolenic acid, an omega-3 fatty acid. Omega-3s help your heart maintain its rhythm, and as a bonus, they may control the pain of rheumatoid arthritis and severe menstrual cramps and fight asthma, breast cancer, and depression. Other vegetable oils provide phytochemicals such as beta-carotene, lutein, and zeaxanthin, all of which fight cancer and protect your eyesight.

You have to use these oils in moderation, though, since they weigh in at 120 calories per tablespoon. If you drench your salad, the increased calories could offset any potential benefits.

Making your own salad dressing can be quicker than you think, and this dressing tastes good and is great for your heart.

Raspberry Dressing

Makes 1 cup

    1   cup fresh or thawed and drained frozen raspberries
    ¼   cup balsamic vinegar
    4   teaspoons olive oil
        Pinch of ground black pepper

Place a fine sieve over a small bowl. Using the back of a spoon, press the raspberries through the sieve to remove the seeds. Add the vinegar, oil, and pepper to the puree and mix to combine.

Per 2 tablespoons: 35 calories, 2.3 g fat (59% of calories), 0.1 g protein, 3.5 g carbohydrates, 0 mg cholesterol, 0.7 g dietary fiber, 1 mg sodium

New Info on Antioxidants

You may have heard some of the hubbub about the antioxidant vitamins C and E and the phytochemical beta-carotene (which converts into vitamin A) and how they don't appear to work as effectively as they were once thought to.

Upon first hearing this news, you might think this would be a strike against vegetables—until you realize that these antioxidants appeared to be ineffective in supplement form. When left as whole foods, the evidence remains strong that vegetables provide an array of heart-healthy benefits.

In fact, as research gets more detailed, scientists are finding additional compounds in vegetables, known as flavonoids, that may help the heart. This is why you may now hear nutrition experts recommend selecting "brightly colored" vegetables, such as dark leafy greens, red peppers, and other bright choices. "The darker the color, the more antioxidants and flavonoids the vegetable has," says Dr. Gardner.

If that isn't enough reason to start eating vegetables, there's still more evidence: Dr. Gardner recently completed a study in which a vegetable-based diet was more effective at lowering cholesterol than the typical low-fat diet. In the study, 59 people with high cholesterol ate a diet that was rich in vegetables, whole grains, soy foods, fruit, beans, and nuts. Another 61 ate a standard low-fat diet that consisted of typical low-fat meats, cheeses, and dressings.

At the end of a 4-week period, both groups saw their total cholesterol and LDL levels fall. But the group eating the plant-based diet saw drops that were almost double the other group's—18 total points, and 14 LDL points, compared to 9 and 7, respectively, for the low-fat diet group. Yet another reason that more vegetables are a great addition to a heart-healthy diet.

A Bumper Crop of Produce Pointers

You don't have to be a vegetarian to appreciate perfectly steamed asparagus or a fresh ear of corn. These strategies can help maximize vegetables' nutrients—and flavors.

• Choose fresh or frozen vegetables over canned; they taste better and contain more nutrients. If you opt for frozen, read the package to make sure the product doesn't contain added salt or fat.

• Steam rather than boil vegetables. They'll be ready in 5 minutes, retain most of their nutrients, and still taste crunchy and delicious.

• Top baked potatoes and steamed vegetables with a blend of fat-free yogurt, garlic, a sprinkling of "light" salt, and a dash each of curry powder and cayenne pepper. Delicious.

• Season vegetables with rice vinegar or another flavored vinegar. This will add bold flavor—without any butter.

• Liven up cooked vegetables with herbs and spices. Some good choices are dill on carrots, chives on a baked potato, garlic and rosemary on fresh green beans, and ginger on sweet potatoes.

• At your next barbecue, pass up the ribs and grill some vegetables. "Marinate sliced eggplant in low-sodium teriyaki sauce, ginger, and garlic, then barbecue it," suggests Janet Lepke-Harris, RD, a dietitian in Charlotte, North Carolina, and a spokesperson for the American Dietetic Association. "It tastes delicious over rice." Try grilling big slices of mushrooms, peppers, and zucchini, too. You can find suitable skewers or racks wherever grill accessories are sold, so food doesn't fall into the coals or burners.

• Want to make a low-fat cream sauce for vegetables? Blend a teaspoon each of low-fat margarine and flour, then heat for 2 minutes while slowly whisking in fat-free milk, suggests Marilyn Cerino, RD, nutrition consultant at the Benjamin Franklin Center for Health of Pennsylvania Hospital in Philadelphia. Add seasonings appropriate to the vegetables.

• Prepare vegetables with flair, says Michael Klaper, MD, health director of the Royal Atlantic Health Spa in Pompano Beach, Florida, and author of *Vegan Nutrition: Pure and Simple.* "You don't have to eat dry, plain vegetables. Have some fun with them. When you make pasta primavera, for example, use lots of green and yellow vegetables. Top rice or noodles with Chinese-style stir-fried vegetables. If you like East Indian cuisine, learn to make a vegetable curry."

• Don't shower vegetables with salt. A high-sodium diet may contribute to high blood pressure, which is no better for your heart than high cholesterol. "Cutting down on salt is like reducing the fat in your diet," says Neal Barnard, MD, president of the Physicians Committee for Responsible Medicine in Washington, D.C. "You get used to it. So squirt a little lemon juice on your broccoli instead of salting it. It can make all the difference in the world."

Vegetarian Diet

Many Options for Going Meatless

If you break down foods into their individual categories, you'll notice a trend develop when it comes to cholesterol—plant foods tend to lower it, and animal foods tend to raise it.

Keeping this basic idea in mind, it would stand to reason that a diet that was *all* plants—such as a vegetarian diet—would lower cholesterol the most. Now that researchers are studying the effects of a vegetarian diet on cholesterol more intensely, that's exactly what appears to be happening. "A number of studies have shown that following a vegetarian diet is more effective at lowering cholesterol than taking prescription statin drugs," says Neal Barnard, MD, president of the Physicians Committee for Responsible Medicine in Washington, D.C.

One of the first to look into this phenomenon was Dean Ornish, MD, president and director of the Preventive Medicine Research Institute in Sausalito, California. In the Lifestyle Heart Trial, he and his colleagues put 28 people with coronary atherosclerosis on a vegetarian diet that derived only 10 percent of its calories from fat. This group also quit smoking, engaged in moderate exercise, and performed stress management techniques such as yoga.

Dr. Ornish compared this group to a different group of 20 people with atherosclerosis who ate a standard diet and took cholesterol-lowering drugs.

After a year, the researchers found that the arteries of 82 percent of the people who followed the low-fat vegetarian diet were less clogged than they had been before the study began. The drug-treatment group ended up with arteries that were more clogged. And—get this—the people whose arteries were the most closed to begin with showed the greatest improvement.

This is by no means the only study that has shown the effectiveness of a vegetarian diet on heart health. Researchers at the University of Toronto have recently completed a number of studies that looked at the Portfolio Eating Plan, a nearly vegan diet that's rich in almonds, oats, barley, soy, plant sterols and stanols, and high-fiber fruits and vegetables. (For more information on this diet, visit www.PortfolioEatingPlan.com.)

After conducting a number of studies about the effects of the diet on people with high cholesterol, the researchers were amazed by the results: Some people in the study lowered their "bad" LDL cholesterol by as much as 35 percent. And when the study went head to head with a group taking cholesterol-lowering statin drugs, the cholesterol-lowering results achieved by the diet matched those of the statins.

One of the most exciting parts of the Portfolio Eating Plan study, though, was that the most recently completed portion of the study showed that the diet does not need to be nearly vegan, or even vegetarian, to achieve good results. When patients were allowed to choose and prepare foods on their own, after being educated about the basic tenets of the Portfolio Eating Plan, one-third of the patients still lowered their LDL cholesterol by 20 percent after a year.

A New Approach to Vegetarianism

The findings of the Portfolio Eating Plan bring to light the new outlook on vegetarianism. Though it was once considered almost counterculture, hard science has now shown that it may be the most effective way to reduce cholesterol and prevent heart disease through diet.

Furthermore, the studies show that even adhering to some vegetarian principles occasionally can help you derive some benefits. By choosing soy instead of meat 3 or 4 days a week, for example, you'll still help your heart more than if you had never selected soy at all.

For those who are concerned about their heart health but hesitant to give up meat completely, this is great news and will certainly be a step in the right

What Kind of Vegetarian Are You?

There are several types of vegetarians, all of whom eat fruits, vegetables, grains, and legumes. But some vegetarians eat dairy products and eggs, while others don't. Some people even qualify as part-time vegetarians, who eat meatless meals made with pastas, beans, and grains several times a week. Here's a rundown of the most common types of vegetarians.

- Semivegetarians eat poultry, fish, and dairy products.

- Lacto-ovo vegetarians eat both dairy products and eggs.

- Lacto vegetarians eat dairy products but not eggs.

- Ovo vegetarians eat eggs but not dairy products.

- Vegans don't eat poultry, fish, dairy products, or eggs.

direction. Of course, if you are ready to take the plunge into full-blown vege-tarianism or veganism, this lifestyle change can have the greatest impact of all.

"If people follow a proper vegan diet, cholesterol becomes a nonissue, as does weight, diabetes, colon cancer, other cancers, hypertension, and oth-ers," says Jeff Popick, an expert on veganism and author of *The Real Forbidden Fruit*. "Before I stopped eating meat and dairy, my cholesterol was over 300. Within a couple of months after becoming vegan, my cholesterol was cut in half. This is a very typical result. In fact, my 'genetics' had me ordained to heart disease, and now I am free of it, simply by following a vegan diet."

The key with a vegetarian or vegan diet is to choose your foods carefully to prevent any deficiencies that can arise from giving up meat. The advice below should help you do exactly that.

Ready for Veggies? Read This First

A vegetarian diet isn't automatically healthy. A steady diet of pizza, potato chips, and chocolate cream pie may satisfy your taste buds, but not your body's need for vitamins and minerals. Here's how to make sure you get the nutrients you need without the fat and cholesterol you don't.

• If you're on a vegetarian diet that allows dairy products, eat the low-fat or fat-free varieties. Whole-milk cheese and whole milk are loaded with saturated fat, which can send your blood cholesterol skyward.

• If you omit all animal products from your diet, you may fall short in pro-tein or vitamin B_{12}. So make sure your diet emphasizes protein-rich plant foods such as beans, peas, and nuts.

  Also, eat cereals fortified with vitamin B_{12} (a nutrient found naturally only in animal foods). If you give up only meat and not eggs or dairy foods, you'll be more likely to get the vitamin B_{12} you need, however.

• If you shun meat, you may also give up plenty of iron, zinc, and calcium. You can get more of these vital nutrients by consuming tofu, beans, peas, and orange juice fortified with calcium.

See also Beans, Fiber, Fruit, Nuts, Oats, Plant Stanols and Sterols, Soy Foods, Vegetables

Walking
The Exercise for Everyone

Think walking isn't intense enough to do your heart any good? The newest research seems to indicate that it might just be the perfect heart-healthy exercise.

In years past, walking often drew criticism for not being as effective as jogging, running, cycling, and other more intense cardiovascular workouts. But a 2007 study shows that more intense cardiovascular exercise might lead to oxidative stress, which means additional wear and tear on the heart and arteries.

Michael Miller, MD, director of preventive cardiology at the University of Maryland Medical Center in Baltimore, conducted the study that led to these discoveries. It all started with a colleague of his who—despite being a marathon runner—had a high buildup of calcium in his coronary arteries. As it turned out, all that intense exercise may have actually contributed to the condition.

Dr. Miller is quick to point out that this individual case should by no means sway people away from exercising, and more study is needed to determine the effects of intense cardiovascular activity on the heart. But it is sufficient evidence to put another feather in the cap of walking as a heart-healthy exercise, says Dr. Miller.

"Over the past few years, it has become clear that moderate activity is cardio-protective," he says. "Brisk walking, in the 3- to 4-mile-per-hour range, provides benefit without significant wear and tear on the joints."

Need more reasons to start walking? Consider this: A number of studies have shown that walking is protective against high cholesterol, high blood pressure, heart attack, stroke, and diabetes.

In addition to the proven health benefits, no exercise is more accessible and convenient to a larger percentage of people than walking is. "Walking is convenient and easy to do and requires no special equipment," says Darlene A. Sedlock, PhD, associate professor of kinesiology at Purdue University in West Lafayette, Indiana. "You can just step out your back door and go."

You may have noticed that the federal government recently increased its exercise guidelines. Currently, 30 minutes a day is the absolute minimum that's recommended: The government says that people should strive for 60 minutes a day to maintain their weight or 90 minutes a day to lose weight or maintain weight loss. That's quite an increase.

If you're a walker, though, it's no problem. Just as walking is convenient and accessible, it's also much easier to sustain for a longer period of time than most other activities—making it the perfect choice for boosting your daily amount of exercise.

Step Lively to Stay Heart Healthy

There's a significant amount of evidence to suggest that walking can promote heart health. Here are a few of those studies.

Investigators at the Cooper Institute in Dallas gave treadmill tests to more than 13,000 people and followed their fitness levels for 8 years. They discovered that folks who walked for a half an hour a day had reduced levels of premature death at almost the same rate as that of people who ran 30 to 40 miles a week.

Researchers at Brigham Young University in Provo, Utah, examined how walking affected the cholesterol levels of more than 3,600 people. The ratios of total cholesterol to HDL cholesterol in folks who walked for 2½ to 4 or more hours per week were less likely to be elevated (a ratio of five or higher) than the ratios of those who didn't exercise regularly.

Regular brisk walking increased "good" HDL cholesterol in 10 sedentary women who took part in a British study. These women (average age 47) followed a walking regimen for 3 months. Not only did brisk walking increase their HDL, but when researchers retested the women after 6 months of not walking, they discovered that the women's cardiovascular gains were lost.

Walking may also help stomp high levels of triglycerides (another blood fat implicated in heart disease) by stimulating an enzyme that carries triglycerides out of the blood, according to researchers at Baylor College of Medicine in Houston. These researchers had one group of 12 people take a single 2-hour walk. A second group didn't exercise at all. Then, 15 hours later, all of the participants ate a high-fat meal. After eating, the walkers' triglyceride readings were 31 percent lower than those of the nonexercisers.

How Fast? How Far?

In 2005, the government concluded that people can gain the most benefit by getting between 60 and 90 minutes of exercise every day. While this is a good idea for everyone, the research has shown that you'll still gain some benefit from walking less or at a slower pace.

Researchers at the Cooper Institute had 59 women walk 3 miles a day, 5 days a week, for 6 months. But each group walked at varying speeds. The first group of women walked a mile in 12 minutes. The second group walked a mile in 15 minutes. And the third group took 20 minutes to walk a mile. The fastest group of women had more impressive improvements in their overall fitness than the slowest group. But the HDL levels of all three groups jumped an average of 6 percent.

As you can see, even if you walk more slowly than others, or can't walk a long distance right away, there are still some very compelling reasons to get out there and hit the pavement!

Ready, Set, Walk!

Ready to start stepping? These expert tips can help you keep pace.

• Invest in a good, comfortable pair of walking shoes. While you don't need hundred-dollar footwear, "you need more than ordinary tennis shoes for walking," says James Rippe, MD, director of the Center for Clinical and Lifestyle Research at Tufts University School of Medicine in Boston and coauthor of *Dr. James Rippe's Complete Book of Fitness Walking*. The shoe you choose should be lightweight and padded at the heel and tongue as well as have an absorbent lining. Also, the shoe should bend easily across the ball of your foot and feature an uptilted sole to enhance your natural walking motion.

• Find a walking buddy. Invite a co-worker to take a "walk break" instead of a coffee break, then take a 15-minute stroll. You might even ask your spouse to share your walk before or after work.

• Walk with the weather in mind. In hot weather, wear loose-fitting, lightweight clothes, advises Dr. Rippe. And try to walk in the early morning or early evening, when the heat is less intense. Drink lots of water before and during your walk.

• In cold weather, dress in light layers that you can easily remove as your body warms up. In truly stormy weather, climb up and down the stairs in your home. *Caution:* If you have heart disease, diabetes, asthma, or other health conditions, consult your doctor before walking in cold weather.

• Join a local walking club. If you can't find one, consider starting your own.

• Forge new paths. Explore the grounds of a nearby botanical garden on foot. Or buy a book of local walking tours and hit the road.

• Imagine success. Visualize yourself on a brisk walk, feeling refreshed, positive, and healthy. After all, a true power walk has just as much to do with the way you feel inside as with the speed of your stride.

See also Exercise

Weight Loss
The Most Basic Way to Lower Cholesterol

Not to revert to clichés, but sometimes lowering cholesterol can be a classic case of not seeing the forest for the trees. Granted, there are a number of foods, activities, and other lifestyle choices that can have an impact on cholesterol. When analyzed individually, each is interesting in its own right— which is why we devoted an entire book to them!

But when you throw out the *specific type* of food, and the *specific type* of activity, one simple fact remains: If you lose weight, your cholesterol will go down. Moreover, lose weight, and you will be reducing your risk of heart disease in multiple ways.

"For many years, excess weight was seen as a contributor to elevated LDL levels, but the relationship was viewed as solely single dimensional—for example, getting to a healthy body weight reduces total cholesterol levels by 5 to 10 percent," says Karen Miller Kovach, RD, chief nutritionist at Weight

Watchers International in Jericho, New York. "The role of excess weight is now seen as a dimension with multiple consequences. Excess weight contributes to several factors, including high blood pressure, high triglycerides, and increased insulin levels and especially waist circumference. By not isolating weight as a single variable, its role in preventing heart disease has escalated considerably."

The impact of obesity on your heart health can be quite substantial. But the good news is, if you can get that weight off and keep it off, your body should be able to turn things around fairly quickly.

Love Handles? Check Your Cholesterol

Numerous studies have made a connection between body weight, elevated cholesterol levels, and risk of coronary heart disease.

Using data from the second National Health and Nutrition Examination Survey, researchers from the University of Texas Southwestern Medical Center at Dallas and other institutions examined the association between excess body weight and high blood cholesterol levels. These researchers conducted two separate studies: one with men, the other with women. Both reached the same conclusion: Excess body weight is associated with higher levels of total and "bad" LDL cholesterol and lower levels of "good" HDL cholesterol in white men and women, whatever their ages.

Perimenopausal and menopausal women had lower HDL cholesterol and higher total and LDL cholesterol than premenopausal women, regardless of their weight. What's more, researchers discovered a stronger connection between body weight and triglyceride levels than between body weight and cholesterol. High levels of triglycerides (another type of blood fat that's implicated in heart disease) are now established as an independent risk factor for coronary heart disease in men and women.

Weigh In for the Last Time

Losing weight is one thing; keeping it off is quite another. But it can be done. These tips can help you shed those pounds permanently.

• Focus on the four pillars. "In order to have a lasting weight loss, four pillars must be in place. They are making wise food choices, engaging in regular physical activity, developing those cognitive skills predictive of maintaining weight loss, and having a supportive environment," says Kovach. "If all four pillars are not in place, the likelihood of long-term weight loss is reduced. Simply paying attention to food choices or activity or a combination of the two is not enough and a key reason why so many people either fail to lose weight or regain it after a loss."

• Work that body. There's no way around it, experts say. "The only way to lose weight is to burn more calories than you consume—not just today or this week, but on a regular basis," says Leonard Doberne, MD, an endocrinologist in Mount View, California.

More important, regular exercise can maintain or even raise HDL cholesterol. While cutting back on dietary fat and cholesterol can often lower total blood cholesterol levels about 15 percent, it also tends to reduce HDL cholesterol, notes Dr. Doberne. "So the ratio of total cholesterol to HDL cholesterol, which appears to be of primary importance, is not always much improved," he says. "Exercise is the best way we know to raise HDL. That's why a weight-loss program aimed at improving the cholesterol ratio should include exercise."

• Avoid crash diets. They tend to slow the metabolism until the body kicks into survival mode and starts storing fat like crazy. Worse, once you start eating normally again, your metabolism is still sluggish, so any pounds you may have lost quickly return.

• Think twice about high-protein diets. People who once devoured pretzels and bagels—both laden with carbohydrates—have given them up in

Eat More at High Noon, Less Later On

It's common knowledge that what we eat affects our weight. But so can *when* we eat it, according to Deepak Chopra, MD, in his book *Perfect Weight*.

According to Ayurveda, the ancient Indian system of natural medicine, the body's "digestive fire" burns strongest at midday. Because digestion is stronger during this time, the body converts food into energy more efficiently, says Dr. Chopra. In fact, many health professionals here in the West suggest eating a bigger breakfast and lunch and a lighter evening meal.

Make lunch your largest meal of the day and eat at approximately the same time each day, preferably between 12:00 and 12:30 p.m., suggests Dr. Chopra. "This one very simple change will make a profound difference in your metabolism," he says.

favor of high-protein foods like beef. These diets are all based on the incorrect notion that carbohydrates make you fat. When people lose weight on a high-protein diet, they think it's because they're eating fewer carbohydrates, but it's really because they're eating fewer calories.

• Cut the fat. Eating fatty foods such as processed lunchmeat, fried snacks, and butter is the fastest route to weight gain. When you consider that fat has 9 calories per gram, or more than twice as many calories as carbohydrates or protein, it's easy to see why fatty foods can lead you to pack on pounds in a hurry.

• Eat more complex carbohydrates—whole grains, legumes, vegetables, and fruits—recommends Deralee Scanlon, RD, manager of professional and consumer education for Pharmavite, a supplement company in Northridge, California, and the author of *Diets That Work.*

Why? Because the body expends more calories digesting and metabolizing complex carbohydrates. To transform 100 calories of carbohydrates into stored body fat, the body must use up 23 calories. But the body uses only 3 calories to convert 100 calories of dietary fat into body fat.

Foods high in complex carbohydrates tend to be higher in fiber and lower in calories and fat. It's likely that these foods also are more filling and take longer to chew—two qualities that can help you reduce the amount you eat.

• Slow down. It takes about 20 minutes for your brain to let your body know that you've eaten enough, says Scanlon. If you eat quickly, you're likely to eat more than you really want.

• Also, before you pick up your fork to begin eating, close your eyes and take a few deep breaths. This can help you eat at a slower, more leisurely pace.

See also Cooking, Exercise, Walking

Whole Grains

The Heart-Smart Carbs

Though much of the rage over the "low-carb/no-carb" diets such as Atkins has finally subsided, the legacy left behind by these diets is a dangerous one: Many people now believe that carbohydrates are bad and are the primary cause of obesity.

This notion is completely false. In reality, carbohydrates are a vital source of energy in every diet. In fact, in the USDA's latest version of the Food Guide Pyramid, carbohydrates are the largest food group to focus on in most people's daily eating plans.

The key is not to avoid carbs, but to choose the *right* carbs. And the right kind of carbohydrates are the complex ones found in whole grains like oats, barley, and whole grain rice, cereal, and pasta, says Deralee Scanlon, RD, manager of professional and consumer education for Pharmavite, a supplement company in Northridge, California, and author of *Diets That Work*.

A Two-Pronged Cholesterol Attack

Whole grains—and the complex carbohydrates found within them—fight cholesterol both directly and indirectly. Directly, whole grains are one of the richest sources of fiber in the diet. Most whole grains have more insoluble fiber (the kind that helps keep you regular) than soluble fiber (the kind that gloms onto cholesterol and flushes it out of the body). Yet one specific whole grain is a soluble fiber superstar: oat bran. Each serving has 4 total grams of fiber, 2 grams of which are soluble fiber.

Though not as heart healthy as soluble fiber, insoluble fiber can play a role in reducing cholesterol. According to Ann G. Kulze, MD, founder and CEO of Just Wellness, a wellness consulting firm in Mt. Pleasant, South Carolina, and the author of *Dr. Ann's 10-Step Diet*, insoluble fiber can improve cholesterol metabolism by enhancing insulin sensitivity. Insulin resistance, which is the opposite of insulin sensitivity, is associated with elevated "bad" LDL cholesterol levels and reduced "good" HDL levels.

Whole grains also have a profound indirect effect on cholesterol by preventing weight gain. When you consider what a great cardiovascular risk excess weight can be, this might even be a more important role for whole grains than their being high in fiber.

Scanlon says that complex carbohydrates help you keep weight off in a few different ways. For one, your body must use more calories to digest and metabolize complex carbohydrates than it does for other foods, which helps you lose more weight. Second, because these foods are higher in fiber and lower in calories and fat, it takes you longer to chew these foods, which makes you eat less. Third, they will make you feel fuller faster, which may keep you from picking up your spoon for another helping. All of these make whole grains a great food for either losing or maintaining weight.

When you consider what foods whole grains typically replace in the diet—namely, the refined carbohydrates found in white bread, snack crackers, and other junk food—their healthy benefits multiply greatly. "Refined carbohydrates like white bread, white potatoes, white rice, and sweets tend to promote insulin resistance, which causes deposition of fat in the liver and abdominal area," says Dr. Kulze. "Fat that accumulates in these areas secretes bioactive substances that elevate bad LDL cholesterol and lower good HDL cholesterol. These foods have also been shown to promote and perpetuate appetite, which increases the risk of weight gain—and weight gain can further increase cholesterol levels. What's more, these foods are largely devoid of beneficial fiber."

As you can see, there are a lot of heart-healthy reasons to choose whole grains over the alternative: refined carbohydrates. Here's what studies have shown about whole grains.

The Hard Science on Whole Grains

Perhaps the most concrete evidence that choosing whole grain foods over refined carbohydrates promotes healthy cholesterol levels comes from a study conducted by Christopher Gardner, PhD, of the Stanford Prevention Research Center at Stanford University Medical Center. In the study, Dr. Gardner and his colleagues divided 120 people into two test groups. One group consumed a typical "American" low-fat diet that was loaded with simple, refined sources of carbohydrates, such as reduced-fat snack foods, reduced-fat salad dressings, potatoes, and other typical low-fat choices you'd see at the grocery store. The second group consumed a diet rich in whole grains, such as oats, brown rice, and soy, as well as plentiful fruits, beans, nuts, and vegetables.

At the end of a 4-week test period, the differences between the two groups were fairly significant. The 59 people who ate the diet with whole grains saw their average total cholesterol fall by 18 points and their LDL drop by 14. For the 61 people in the "low-fat" group, total cholesterol fell by an average of 9 points, and LDL fell 7 points. Dr. Gardner cited the inclusion of whole grains, beans, nuts, and produce as the main reason for the difference in cholesterol readings between the two groups.

This is by no means the only example of a diet using whole grains to lower cholesterol. In a separate study at the University of Toronto, a diet that included whole grains like soy, oats, and barley—along with other healthy foods like almonds and margarine with plant stanols and sterols—lowered cholesterol almost as much as prescription cholesterol-lowering statin drugs. After 1 month, the group of patients taking the statins saw their LDL cholesterol drop by 30.9 percent, while the group eating the special diet saw a drop of 28.6 percent—pretty convincing proof that whole grains are a vital part of a heart-healthy diet.

Filling the "Whole"

Trying to fill up on whole grains in your own diet? It's easier now than it ever has been. "One of the simplest ways that you can boost fiber is transitioning from refined carbohydrates to their whole grain counterparts," says Dr. Kulze. "And you can find ultimately every imaginable bread product—including bagels, English muffins, pizza dough, and crackers—in a 100 percent whole grain version now. Just making this switch alone will help you decrease LDL cholesterol levels and raise HDL levels."

Here are some other ways to get more grains in your diet.

• Look for ways to add whole grains to "medley"-style dishes. Barley, for example, is quite good in vegetable soup, and bulgur wheat works well in a casserole or a stir-fry.

• In pancakes, waffles, muffins, or other flour-based recipes, try using whole grain or oat flour for up to half of the regular flour. It may increase the leavening time and the dough's density somewhat, but you can experiment with gradually increasing the amount of whole grain flour until you get the texture just right.

• Use oats or whole grain cereal as breading for baked chicken, fish, or eggplant.

- Choose popcorn, whole grain cereal, or baked whole grain tortilla chips as snacks.
- If you're going to make cookies, always add some oatmeal to the batter.

See also Weight Loss

Yogurt
A Great Alternative to High-Fat Dairy

Yogurt is the classic case of a food helping out your heart by indirect means. While it doesn't specifically lower blood cholesterol, yogurt is so versatile that it can be used in your diet in a variety of ways to replace high-fat, heart-clogging fare.

The key, as with other dairy products, is to choose low-fat or fat-free yogurt over the whole-milk varieties. You'll find that they taste every bit as good as their whole-milk counterparts. What's more, yogurt is a rich source of calcium, which not only is good for your bones but also has been shown in a number of studies to reduce cholesterol. A cup of yogurt has roughly 300 to 450 milligrams of calcium—more than a glass of milk and enough to meet one-third to one-half of most people's daily requirements.

Pick a fruit-flavored yogurt for a great snack on its own or for a side dish or dessert for your favorite meal. Plain yogurt is even more versatile, as it's a great stand-in for higher-fat dairy foods in recipes. (See some great ideas for using plain yogurt below.)

If you're looking for even more reasons to add yogurt to your heart-healthy regimen, it's a rich source of protein and B vitamins. Plus, it's low in lactose, a milk sugar that prevents many people from enjoying dairy products. So it's a great way for people with lactose intolerance to get the benefits of dairy safely.

Dips, Desserts, and More

Whether you're craving a savory dip or a succulent dessert, yogurt can help fit the bill—deliciously. Try these suggestions.

• Top pancakes and waffles with low-fat or fat-free fruit-flavored yogurt instead of butter and syrup.

• For a tasty breakfast treat, stir a few tablespoons of wheat germ or high-fiber cereal into a cup of fat-free vanilla yogurt.

• To make a deliciously different dressing for chicken salad, blend low-fat or fat-free vanilla yogurt with fat-free mayonnaise, suggests Marilyn Cerino, RD, nutrition consultant at the Benjamin Franklin Center for Health of Pennsylvania Hospital in Philadelphia.

• Create a creamy dip for raw vegetables or other low-fat snacks by mixing fat-free yogurt with fat-free sour cream, dill, and garlic, says Janet Lepke-Harris, RD, a dietitian in Charlotte, North Carolina, and a spokesperson for the American Dietetic Association.

• Substitute fat-free plain yogurt for sour cream or buttermilk in home-made baked goods. "Drain the yogurt through a piece of cheesecloth or a coffee filter," suggests Cerino. "You'll end up with a nice, thick product that you can add to muffins and quick breads."

• Jazz up plain or vanilla yogurt with some chopped fresh fruit.

• Whip up a frothy yogurt smoothie by blending fat-free plain or vanilla yogurt with fresh fruit or juice.

• If you're an ice cream maven, enjoy low-fat or fat-free frozen yogurt rather than premium ice cream. You'll save yourself 30 or more grams of fat. It's possible to have too much of a good thing, however, and low-fat treats are no exception. So make sure you don't overdo it.

Most people with diabetes can eat foods that contain artificial sweeteners, like some fruit-flavored yogurts. But if you are pregnant and have diabetes (gestational diabetes), it's a good idea to avoid products flavored with these substances just to be on the safe side. Instead, choose plain yogurt and mix in some fresh fruit.

See also Calcium

PART TWO

The Breakthrough Menu Plan

Cut Cholesterol 30 Points in 30 Days

Want to gorge on three squares (plus snacks) a day and lower your cholesterol 30 points in 30 days? Have we got a meal plan for you!

This nutritionist-approved menu plan, which was designed to lower cholesterol 30 points in 30 days, provides about 2,000 calories a day, with 55 percent of calories from complex carbohydrates (starches), 20 percent from fat, 15 percent from protein, and 10 percent from simple carbohydrates (sugars). And of the 20 percent of calories from fat, only about 5 percent come from saturated fat. The typical U.S. diet contains 13 percent of calories from saturated fat.

As for cholesterol, this plan includes 150 milligrams a day, which is half of the American Heart Association's recommended limit of 300 milligrams a day. The plan also contains more fiber and less sodium than the typical U.S. diet. All meals provide one serving.

To reduce your cholesterol 30 points in 30 days, you have to switch from the typical American diet (which gets about 37 percent of its calories from fat) to the diet outlined in the following pages—and follow it to the letter. If you eat 30 percent of calories from fat, for example, your cholesterol may drop about 15 points in 30 days.

But if you think lowering your cholesterol while enjoying tasty, filling meals sounds too good to be true, you're in for a pleasant surprise. This is a diet that anyone can follow—and enjoy!

Menu plan: Anita Hirsch, RD, former nutritionist, Rodale Test Kitchen.

Menu plan review: Sonja L. Connor, RD, research associate professor of clinical nutrition at the Oregon Health Sciences University in Portland.

Day 1

Breakfast

¾ cup grape juice

1 cup oatmeal with ¼ cup raisins and ¼ cup fat-free milk

⅛ wedge cantaloupe

Lunch

1 cup cooked pasta with ½ cup low-sodium marinara sauce

Tossed salad: 1 cup chopped romaine lettuce, ½ cup shredded carrots, and ½ cup shredded red cabbage, dressed with 2 teaspoons canola oil, 2 tablespoons vinegar, and a dash of sweet basil

Garlic bread: 2 slices toasted Italian bread, brushed with 2 teaspoons olive oil and rubbed with 1 clove fresh garlic

Dinner

Fresh vegetable platter: ¼ cup cauliflower, ¼ green pepper, sliced, and ¼ cup chopped mushrooms

Vegetable dip: ¼ cup fat-free yogurt, flavored with 1 scallion, chopped

3 ounces broiled haddock

¾ cup steamed rice

1 cup steamed broccoli with ¼ teaspoon fresh ginger or a dash of dried ginger

½ cup cubed winter squash and ¼ cup crushed pineapple, sprinkled with nutmeg

Snacks

2 ounces fat-free unsalted pretzels

1 apple, sliced and topped with ½ cup low-fat vanilla yogurt, 2 teaspoons wheat germ, and 1 tablespoon slivered almonds

Daily totals: 1,932 calories, 34 g total fat, 3.6 g saturated fat, 65 mg cholesterol, 30 g dietary fiber, 1,457 mg sodium

Day 2

Breakfast

½ English muffin with 1 tablespoon strawberry spread and 1 teaspoon diet margarine

½ cup low-fat vanilla yogurt with 2 tablespoons wheat germ

1 orange

Lunch

1 cup grape juice

Turkey sandwich: 1 ounce white meat turkey on 2 slices whole wheat bread with lettuce, tomato, and 1 teaspoon mustard

Tossed salad: 3 cups chopped greens, 1 carrot, sliced, and ¼ cup chickpeas, dressed with 2 teaspoons olive oil and 2 tablespoons flavored vinegar

4 graham crackers

Dinner

1 cup low-sodium minestrone soup

3 ounces lean roast beef

1 baked potato, topped with butter-flavored sprinkles and a dash of garlic powder

½ cup steamed brussels sprouts, topped with 1 tablespoon vinegar and a dash of dry mustard

2 slices Italian bread with 2 teaspoons diet margarine

1 cup canned peaches, in juice

Snacks

½ bagel with 1 tablespoon low-fat cream cheese

1 pear

Daily totals: 1,982 calories, 36 g total fat, 9 g saturated fat, 96 mg cholesterol, 38 g dietary fiber, 1,796 mg sodium

Day 3

Breakfast

¾ cup orange juice

1 cup ready-to-eat raisin bran cereal with ½ cup fat-free milk

2 dried figs

Lunch

Vegetable burger on whole wheat bun with lettuce, tomato, onion, and mustard

½ cup commercially prepared three-bean salad

1 carrot and 1 stalk celery, cut into sticks

½ cup low-fat coffee-flavored yogurt

1 tangerine or other fresh fruit

Dinner

Tossed salad: 3 cups chopped romaine lettuce, 2 slices tomato, ½ carrot, sliced, 2 radishes, and 2 slices cucumber, dressed with 2 teaspoons olive oil and 2 tablespoons vinegar

3 ounces grilled or baked chicken breast, rubbed with fresh garlic and ½ teaspoon olive oil

1 cup steamed brown rice

Savory cabbage: ½ cup shredded cabbage and ¼ cup chopped onions, sautéed in 2 teaspoons olive oil, ½ teaspoon savory, and ½ teaspoon dill

1 baked apple with 2 tablespoons maple syrup

Snacks

3 fat-free devil's food cookies

2 cups air-popped popcorn with ½ teaspoon butter-flavored sprinkles

Daily totals: 1,969 calories, 38 g total fat, 8.6 g saturated fat, 95 mg cholesterol, 39 g dietary fiber, 1,909 mg sodium

Day 4

Breakfast

1½ cups ready-to-eat multigrain cereal with ½ cup fat-free milk, sprinkled with 5 almonds, chopped

½ red grapefruit

Lunch

1 cup low-sodium split pea soup

1 toasted English muffin with 2 teaspoons diet margarine

¾ cup low-fat or fat-free strawberry yogurt with 1 teaspoon rice bran or wheat germ

Dinner

Pork stir-fry: 1 ounce lean pork loin, 1 cup sliced bok choy, ½ cup snow peas, ¼ cup diced red peppers, and ¼ cup diced celery, stir-fried in 1 teaspoon minced fresh garlic, 2 teaspoons canola oil, and a dash of sesame oil

1½ cups steamed brown rice with a dash of poultry seasoning or sage

Tossed salad: 1 cup shredded romaine lettuce, ¼ cup chopped red onions, and 2 radishes, dressed with 1 tablespoon lemon juice and 2 teaspoons olive oil

1 banana or other fresh fruit

Snacks

1 cup grapes

1 bake-and-eat soft pretzel (2½ ounces, baked without salt)

Daily totals: 1,941 calories, 40 g total fat, 6.8 g saturated fat, 33 mg cholesterol, 25 g dietary fiber, 1,465 mg sodium

Day 5

Breakfast

1 English muffin with 2 teaspoons diet margarine

Breakfast blender drink: 1 cup fat-free milk and ½ cup fresh or unsweetened frozen strawberries, blended until frothy

Lunch

Pita sandwich: 1 ounce cubed low-fat Cheddar cheese, ½ cup chopped spinach, tomato, and onion, stuffed in a pita and dressed with 2 tablespoons fat-free dressing (your choice)

1 carrot and 1 stalk celery, cut into sticks

1 cup low-fat yogurt (your choice)

Dinner

2 slices pizza (ask for only half the cheese)

Tossed salad: 3 cups chopped greens, ¼ cup broccoli, ¼ cup chickpeas, ¼ tomato, sliced, and 1 tablespoon chopped onions, dressed with 2 tablespoons fat-free dressing (your choice)

1 cup grapes

Snacks

2 cups cooked pasta with ½ cup low-sodium marinara sauce

2 unsalted pretzels (2 ounces)

1 banana

Daily totals: 1,899 calories, 28 g total fat, 7 g saturated fat, 50 mg cholesterol, 26 g dietary fiber, 2,473 mg sodium

Day 6

Breakfast

¾ cup orange juice

Egg substitute, scrambled with 1 tablespoon fat-free milk in a nonstick pan

1 potato, sliced and sautéed with 1 tablespoon diet margarine, 2 tablespoons chopped onions, and ½ clove fresh garlic, minced, in a nonstick pan

2 slices toasted whole wheat bread with 2 teaspoons fruit spread

Lunch

1 cup low-sodium lentil soup

Tossed salad: 3 cups chopped greens, ½ cup sliced carrots, and ¼ cup sliced onions, dressed with 2 teaspoons olive oil and 1 tablespoon vinegar

1 toasted English muffin

Dinner

Chicken fajita: 3 ounces chicken strips (prepared in a low-fat manner), ¼ cup mashed avocado, ¼ cup salsa, ¼ cup fat-free plain yogurt, 1½ teaspoons olive oil, 1 teaspoon lime juice, and 1 teaspoon fresh cilantro in 1 flour tortilla

1½ cups steamed brown rice, flavored with 2 tablespoons salsa and ⅛ teaspoon chopped jalapeño peppers

10 low-fat tortilla chips (1 ounce)

Snacks

1 cup fresh or canned chunked pineapple, in juice

1 carrot, cut into sticks, with ¼ cup commercially prepared fat-free herbed yogurt cheese

Daily totals: 1,902 calories, 45 g total fat, 7.3 g saturated fat, 77 mg cholesterol, 29 g dietary fiber, 1,717 mg sodium

Day 7

Breakfast

½ bagel with 1 tablespoon light cream cheese

1 cup low-fat vanilla yogurt with 2 teaspoons wheat germ

½ mango, cubed

Lunch

2 ounces scallops, ½ cup chopped mushrooms, ¼ cup sliced onions, ¼ cup chopped celery, and ¼ cup chopped green peppers, sautéed with 1 teaspoon sesame oil, 1 tablespoon low-sodium soy sauce, 1 clove fresh garlic, minced, and 1 teaspoon grated fresh ginger

2 cups steamed rice

1 fortune cookie

Dinner

2 cups low-sodium vegetable soup

Tossed salad: 1 ounce flaked water-packed tuna, 4 cups chopped romaine lettuce, ¼ cup shredded carrots, and 1 radish, dressed with 1 teaspoon olive oil and 1 tablespoon vinegar

Baked pita crisps: 1 pita, brushed with 2 teaspoons olive oil and assorted herbs and spices, broiled and broken into pieces

1 cup fresh fruit (grapes, apples, and oranges)

Snacks

2 graham crackers with 1 tablespoon peanut butter and 1 cup fat-free milk

1 banana

Daily totals: 2,030 calories, 40 g total fat, 10 g saturated fat, 61 mg cholesterol, 25 g dietary fiber, 1,761 mg sodium

Day 8

Breakfast

$^3/_4$ cup orange juice

1 cup oatmeal with $^1/_4$ cup raisins and $^1/_2$ cup fat-free milk

1 slice toasted whole wheat bread with 1 teaspoon diet margarine and 1 tablespoon apple butter

Lunch

1 cup low-sodium tomato soup

$^1/_4$ to $^1/_2$ cup commercially prepared three-bean salad (add $^1/_4$ cup chopped red onions, basil, and 2 tablespoons red wine vinegar)

2 slices rye bread with 2 teaspoons diet margarine

1 peach, nectarine, or other fresh fruit

Dinner

Bulgur salad: 1 cup cooked bulgur, 2 tablespoons parsley, $^1/_2$ tomato, chopped, and 1 teaspoon lemon juice

Broiled skinless chicken breast

1 potato, baked, with 2 tablespoons fat-free sour cream and 2 teaspoons diet margarine

1 cup chopped spinach, sautéed in 1 teaspoon olive oil, $^1/_4$ cup chopped onions, and 1 clove fresh garlic, minced

1 hard roll (2 ounces) with 1 tablespoon diet margarine

2 cups cubed watermelon or other fruit

Snacks

2 cups air-popped popcorn with butter-flavored sprinkles and 1 teaspoon Parmesan cheese

1 fresh fig

Daily totals: 1,968 calories, 41 g total fat, 7 g saturated fat, 84 mg cholesterol, 41 g dietary fiber, 1,850 mg sodium

Day 9

Breakfast

$^3/_4$ cup ready-to-eat fortified oat cereal with $^1/_2$ cup fat-free milk

1 sliced banana

Lunch

1 oat bran and raisin muffin (2 ounces)

1 cup low-fat yogurt (your choice)

1 orange, sliced

Dinner

1 cup low-sodium vegetable soup (add $^1/_4$ cup white beans and 1 clove fresh garlic, minced, if desired)

3 ounces baked flounder

$^1/_4$ cup chopped cabbage, sautéed in 2 teaspoons canola oil and ground red pepper (to taste) and served over 1 cup steamed rice

1 slice cornbread with 2 teaspoons diet margarine

1 baked apple with $^1/_2$ teaspoon cinnamon and 2 teaspoons brown sugar

Snacks

6 graham crackers with 1 tablespoon almond butter or peanut butter

$^1/_2$ cup fat-free milk

Daily totals: 1,748 calories, 33 g total fat, 4 g saturated fat, 68 mg cholesterol, 31 g dietary fiber, 1,273 mg sodium

Day 10

Breakfast

1 cup cooked oat bran cereal with 1 tablespoon rice bran or wheat germ

2 cups cubed honeydew, casaba, or other melon

Lunch

1 applesauce muffin (1 ounce) with 2 teaspoons diet margarine

½ cup 2% cottage cheese with 2 cups fresh fruit (your choice)

Dinner

1 cup low-sodium vegetable juice

1 cup low-sodium green pea soup

Spinach salad: 2 cups spinach, ¼ cup sliced mushrooms, ¼ cup chopped red onions, and 1 clove fresh garlic, minced, dressed with 2 teaspoons olive oil and 2 tablespoons vinegar

4 garlic breadsticks (4 ounces)

Snacks

2 fig bars

1 orange

Fresh vegetable plate: 1 cup carrot sticks and ½ cup broccoli florets

Vegetable dip: 2 tablespoons commercially prepared fat-free herbed yogurt cheese

Daily totals: 1,796 calories, 41 g total fat, 11 g saturated fat, 10 mg cholesterol, 44 g dietary fiber, 1,985 mg sodium

Day 11

Breakfast

1 cup hot cereal with 1 tablespoon wheat germ and
2 tablespoons maple syrup

Fruit compote: 2 tablespoons prunes, 2 tablespoons figs,
and 2 tablespoons raisins, cooked in 2 tablespoons orange
juice and 2 tablespoons water

Lunch

1 cup low-sodium turkey vegetable soup

Tossed salad: 4 cups chopped romaine lettuce, dressed
with 2 teaspoons olive oil and 2 tablespoons vinegar

2 slices toasted whole wheat bread

1 cup low-fat yogurt (your choice)

Dinner

3 ounces pork medallions in tomato sauce, served over
1 cup egg noodles

1½ cups steamed green beans and chopped carrots

2 slices rye bread with 2 teaspoons diet margarine

Streusel apple: 1 apple, baked with 1 tablespoon low-fat flavored yogurt, ½ tablespoon oats, and 1 teaspoon brown
sugar

Snack

2 ounces low-sodium pretzel chips with mustard

*Daily totals: 1,996 calories, 41 g total fat, 7.2 g saturated fat,
122 mg cholesterol, 32 g dietary fiber, 1,721 mg sodium*

Day 12

Breakfast

1 cup ready-to-eat bran cereal with $\frac{1}{2}$ cup fat-free milk

2 slices toasted whole wheat bread with 2 teaspoons diet margarine

1 banana

Lunch

$\frac{1}{2}$ grapefruit

Pasta salad: 1 cup cooked pasta, 1 ounce water-packed tuna, $\frac{1}{2}$ cup snow peas, $\frac{1}{2}$ cup frozen or canned plain artichoke hearts, and 2 scallions, chopped, dressed with 1 tablespoon low-fat mayonnaise, 1 tablespoon vinegar, fresh basil and parsley

1 slice pumpernickel bread with 2 teaspoons diet margarine

Dinner

Chicken kebabs: 2 ounces cooked cubed chicken breast with $\frac{1}{4}$ pepper, chunked, $\frac{1}{2}$ tomato, chunked, 5 mushrooms, chunked, and $\frac{1}{3}$ onion, chunked, marinated in 2 teaspoons olive oil, 2 teaspoons lemon juice, 2 teaspoons low-sodium soy sauce, 1 tablespoon chopped parsley, 1 clove fresh garlic, minced, $\frac{1}{4}$ chile pepper, minced, and $\frac{1}{4}$ teaspoon red-pepper flakes

$1\frac{1}{2}$ cups steamed brown and wild rice, tossed with thyme or parsley

1 frozen fruit bar

Snacks

1 cup grapes

1 oat bran and raisin muffin (2 ounces)

Daily totals: 1,895 calories, 33 g total fat, 5 g saturated fat, 65 mg cholesterol, 38 g dietary fiber, 2,065 mg sodium

Day 13

Breakfast

Four 4-inch buckwheat pancakes with 4 tablespoons maple syrup

Citrus salad: ¼ cup grapefruit sections and ½ cup orange sections

Lunch

Egg drop soup: 1 cup hot low-fat chicken stock with 2 tablespoons egg substitute

Chicken teriyaki with vegetables (low-fat, low-calorie frozen entrée)

1½ cups steamed brown rice with chives

Wonton chips: 3 wonton wrappers, misted with nonstick cooking spray and baked

3 kumquats or ½ cup fresh or canned chunked pineapple, in juice

Dinner

Omelet: ⅓ cup chopped mushrooms and ⅓ cup chopped onions, sautéed in 2 teaspoons olive oil and folded into ½ cup beaten egg substitute

2 slices toasted whole wheat bread with 2 teaspoons diet margarine and 1 tablespoon strawberry spread

1 apple, sliced, with 1 tablespoon natural peanut butter

Snacks

1 carrot, cut into sticks

2 slices melba toast with 1-ounce chunk low-fat Swiss cheese

Daily totals: 1,805 calories, 42 g total fat, 11.4 g saturated fat, 123 mg cholesterol, 32 g dietary fiber, 1,978 mg sodium

Day 14

Breakfast

¾ cup tropical fruit juice

2 whole grain waffles, topped with ½ cup low-fat yogurt (your choice) and ½ cup blueberries

Lunch

Turkey sandwich: 1 ounce low-fat turkey breast lunchmeat and 1 ounce low-fat Swiss cheese on 2 slices rye bread with lettuce, tomato, and 2 teaspoons mustard

1 carrot, cut into sticks

Curry dip: ¼ cup fat-free plain yogurt and ¼ cup fat-free mayonnaise, blended with ½ teaspoon curry powder and 1 clove fresh garlic, minced

Dinner

3 ounces boneless, skinless chicken breast, poached with ¼ cup chopped onions, ¼ cup chopped carrots, and 1 tablespoon parsley and served over 1 cup steamed chopped spinach

Hawaiian rice: 1 cup cooked brown rice with ½ cup snow peas, 4 pieces baby corn, and ¼ cup water chestnuts, sautéed in 1 teaspoon peanut oil and ¼ teaspoon ground red pepper and tossed with ¼ cup drained chunked pineapple

1 sweet potato, baked or steamed (top with cinnamon, if desired)

½ mango, sprinkled with ¼ cup macadamia nuts

Snack

1 slice cocoa angel food cake (¹⁄₁₂ cake) with ½ cup fresh raspberries

Daily totals: 2,108 calories, 53 g total fat, 11 g saturated fat, 101 mg cholesterol, 37 g dietary fiber, 2,228 mg sodium

Day 15

Breakfast

1 peach bran muffin (2 ounces)

1 cup fat-free milk

1 pear

Lunch

1 cup low-sodium vegetable soup (add ¼ cup diced carrots and ¼ cup chopped kale, if desired)

Tossed salad: 2 cups chopped greens, 2 tablespoons chopped cabbage, and ¼ cup diced celery, dressed with ¼ cup fat-free yogurt blended with 1 clove fresh garlic, minced

2 slices whole wheat bread with 1 tablespoon natural peanut butter

1 cup grapes

Dinner

2 ounces sliced lean roast beef

Mushroom barley: ⅓ cup chopped mushrooms, sautéed in 2 teaspoons olive oil and ¼ teaspoon thyme and added to 1 cup cooked barley

1 cup steamed sliced carrots

1 slice Italian bread with 1 teaspoon diet margarine

½ cup peaches with ½ cup pureed strawberry sauce

Snacks

1 bake-and-eat soft pretzel (2½ ounces, baked without salt)

1 apple, sliced and sprinkled with cinnamon

Daily totals: 1,895 calories, 40 g total fat, 9 g saturated fat, 108 mg cholesterol, 49 g dietary fiber, 1,666 mg sodium

Day 16

Breakfast

1 English muffin with 2 teaspoons diet margarine, 1 table-spoon fruit spread, and 1 teaspoon wheat germ

1 orange

Lunch

1 potato, baked, with chives and 2 tablespoons fat-free sour cream

Spinach salad: 2 cups chopped spinach, $\frac{1}{2}$ carrot, chopped, $\frac{1}{4}$ cup chopped mushrooms, and $\frac{1}{4}$ cup chopped onions, dressed with 2 tablespoons low-fat dressing (your choice)

2 slices Italian bread with 1 tablespoon diet margarine

Dinner

3 ounces grilled snapper

$\frac{1}{2}$ cup black beans with 4 tablespoons tomato salsa, served over 1 cup steamed rice

1 cup zucchini, sautéed in 2 teaspoons olive oil with $\frac{1}{4}$ cup chopped onions and 1 clove fresh garlic, minced

$\frac{1}{2}$ cup fresh blueberries and $\frac{1}{4}$ cup fat-free vanilla yogurt

Snacks

2 oatmeal cookies (1 ounce each) with 1 cup fat-free milk

2 cups cubed watermelon

Daily totals: 1,809 calories, 34 g total fat, 5.5 g saturated fat, 39 mg cholesterol, 30 g dietary fiber, 1,823 mg sodium

Day 17

Breakfast

¾ cup orange juice

1 cup cooked bulgur with ¼ cup apricot nectar, 1 tablespoon chopped dried fruit bits, ¼ cup fat-free milk, and 2 teaspoons oat bran

Lunch

1 cup low-sodium vegetable soup

Roast beef sandwich: 1 ounce sliced lean roast beef on a hard roll (2 ounces) with romaine lettuce, onion, and 2 teaspoons mustard

Fresh veggie plate: 1 cup cauliflower florets, 1 carrot, cut into sticks, and 2 or 3 cherry tomatoes

2 tablespoons fat-free dressing (your choice)

Dinner

Cheese and spinach lasagna (low-fat frozen entrée)

1 cup steamed broccoli with ¼ teaspoon basil

Garlic bread: 2 slices toasted Italian bread, brushed with 2 teaspoons olive oil and rubbed with 1 clove fresh garlic

Fruit plate: 1 kiwifruit, sliced, and 3 strawberries, sliced

2 reduced-fat cookies

Snacks

2 cups air-popped popcorn with ¼ teaspoon of your choice of seasonings: curry powder, Worcestershire sauce, Parmesan cheese, dill, or butter-flavored sprinkles

1 peach or other seasonal fruit

Daily totals: 1,726 calories, 34 g total fat, 6.7 g saturated fat, 27 mg cholesterol, 32 g dietary fiber, 2,212 mg sodium

Day 18

Breakfast

¾ cup grape juice

1 large shredded-wheat biscuit with ½ cup fat-free milk

1 oat bran and blueberry muffin

Lunch

1 cup low-sodium Manhattan clam chowder

1 slice toasted whole wheat bread, topped with 1 ounce low-fat, low-sodium Cheddar cheese, ¼ cup sliced onions, and 1 slice tomato and broiled

Tossed salad: 2 cups chopped greens, ¼ cup chopped mushrooms, and ¼ cup shredded carrots, dressed with 2 tablespoons low-fat dressing (your choice)

½ cup fresh pineapple wedges

Dinner

2-ounce chicken burger patty on a bun (1 ounce) with lettuce, tomato, and onion

Oven fries: 1 potato, thinly sliced and baked with garlic powder, Italian seasoning, or other spices

1 cup canned or homemade baked beans, without salt

½ cup applesauce with a dash of cinnamon

Snacks

½ cup low-fat frozen yogurt (your choice)

1 bake-and-eat soft pretzel (2½ ounces, baked without salt)

3 vanilla wafers

Daily totals: 1,939 calories, 29 g total fat, 8.5 g saturated fat, 103 mg cholesterol, 46 g dietary fiber, 2,203 mg sodium

Day 19

Breakfast

1 cup cooked oatmeal with 2 teaspoons rice bran and
½ cup fat-free milk

1 orange

Lunch

Tacos: 1 ounce extra-lean ground beef, 8 tablespoons
cooked lentils, 3 tablespoons stewed tomatoes, ¼ tomato,
chopped, ½ cup chopped lettuce, ½ ounce shredded low-
sodium, low-fat Cheddar cheese, 2 tablespoons mashed
avocado, and 2 tablespoons fat-free sour cream, layered
in 2 taco shells

1 cup steamed rice (add 2 tablespoons salsa, if desired)

Dinner

Beef stew: 2 ounces lean beef (bottom round), simmered
in 1 cup water with 1 cup chunked carrots, 1 cup chunked
potatoes, ½ cup sliced onions, 1 clove fresh garlic, minced,
2 tablespoons parsley, 1 teaspoon basil, and 1 teaspoon
savory

1 cup cooked barley or barley/rice mix, flavored with
¼ teaspoon marjoram, ¼ teaspoon chopped onions, and
¼ teaspoon garlic powder

1 slice whole wheat bread or low-sodium cornbread with
2 teaspoons diet margarine

Snacks

1 apple

2 ounces unsalted pretzels

2 cups air-popped popcorn with butter-flavored sprinkles

*Daily totals: 1,870 calories, 31 g total fat, 8 g saturated fat,
84 mg cholesterol, 40 g dietary fiber, 737 mg sodium*

Day 20

Breakfast

1 toasted bagel with 2 tablespoons fat-free cream cheese

1 baked apple with 1 teaspoon diet margarine and 1 table-spoon maple syrup

Lunch

Tossed salad: 2 cups chopped greens with ¼ cup shred-ded carrots, ¼ cup diced celery, ¼ cup shredded cab-bage, ¼ cup frozen or canned plain artichoke hearts, and 1 tablespoon ground chile pepper (if desired), dressed with 2 tablespoons fat-free dressing (your choice)

6 whole wheat crackers

1 cup fresh strawberries or other seasonal fruit

Dinner

Greek salad: 4 cups chopped romaine lettuce, 1 ounce feta cheese, ¼ cup sliced mushrooms, ¼ cup chickpeas, and 2 olives, dressed with 2 tablespoons lemon juice and 1 tablespoon olive oil

3 ounces haddock fillet

1 potato, chunked and roasted with 1 teaspoon rosemary

Ratatouille: ¼ cup tomato sauce, ½ cup chopped egg-plant, ¼ tomato, chopped, ½ zucchini, sliced, and ¼ cup chopped celery, served over ½ cup cooked orzo

¼ cup hummus, spread over 1 pita

½ cup rice pudding with raisins

Snacks

2 fresh or dried figs

½ cup fat-free yogurt (your choice)

1 orange

Daily totals: 1,940 calories, 44 g total fat, 8.5 g saturated fat, 81 mg cholesterol, 42 g dietary fiber, 2,486 mg sodium

Day 21

Breakfast

1 cup oatmeal with ½ cup sliced strawberries, 1 tablespoon brown sugar, and ½ cup fat-free milk

2 slices toasted whole wheat bread with 2 teaspoons diet margarine

Lunch

Pizza: ¼ ready-made pizza crust, ¼ cup tomato sauce, 1 ounce reduced-fat mozzarella cheese, ¼ cup roasted red peppers, ½ teaspoon olive oil, ½ teaspoon hot-pepper flakes, ¼ cup chopped green peppers, ¼ cup chopped red peppers, ¼ cup cooked white beans, and ¼ cup chopped spinach

1 carrot, cut into sticks

½ cup grapes

Dinner

3 ounces lamb (loin chop)

Potato sauté: 1 potato, sliced, ¼ cup chopped mushrooms, ¼ cup chopped onions, 1 tablespoon parsley, and 1 clove fresh garlic, minced, sautéed in ½ cup chicken stock

1 cup steamed brussels sprouts, seasoned with herbes de Provence, savory, or lemon juice

1 roll (2 ounces) with 2 teaspoons diet margarine

1 poached peach, sliced, with nutmeg and cinnamon

Snacks

2 slices toasted cinnamon raisin bread

4 fig bars

Daily totals: 1,881 calories, 39 g total fat, 10 g saturated fat, 98 mg cholesterol, 29 g dietary fiber, 2,012 mg sodium

Day 22

Breakfast

¾ cup orange juice

1 cup ready-to-eat oat cereal with ½ cup fat-free milk

1 banana, sliced

Lunch

1 cup chicken chow mein (low-calorie frozen entrée)

2 cups steamed white rice

1 fortune cookie or fresh fruit

Dinner

3 ounces baked orange roughy

1 cup barley, topped with ½ cup chopped mushrooms and ¼ cup sliced onions sautéed in 2 teaspoons olive oil and ½ cup tomato salsa

1 cup steamed cauliflower

Snacks

1 whole grain waffle, topped with ½ cup frozen yogurt (your choice) and 2 tablespoons chocolate syrup

1 peach, sliced

Daily totals: 1,868 calories, 23 g total fat, 6 g saturated fat, 66 mg cholesterol, 27 g dietary fiber, 1,589 mg sodium

Day 23

Breakfast

1 bagel, topped with 2 tablespoons fat-free cream cheese mixed with 1 tablespoon chopped dates

1 orange

Lunch

Salmon salad: 2 ounces canned red salmon, arranged on 2 cups chopped romaine lettuce with 1 green onion, thinly sliced, and ¼ cup chopped mushrooms and dressed with 2 teaspoons olive oil and 2 tablespoons vinegar

Cucumber and onion salad, dressed with ¼ cup fat-free plain yogurt and dill

Garlic bread: 2 slices toasted Italian bread, brushed with 2 teaspoons olive oil and rubbed with 1 clove fresh garlic

Dinner

1 cup light cheese tortellini

½ cup tomato sauce

½ cup steamed green beans, flavored with ⅛ teaspoon olive oil, fresh rosemary, grated lemon rind, and butter-flavored sprinkles

3 soft breadsticks (1½ ounces total) with 2 teaspoons diet margarine

Mini fruit salad: ½ cup sliced apples and ¼ cup grapes, drizzled with ½ cup low-fat vanilla yogurt

Snacks

Pronto pinto dip: ½ cup cooked pinto beans, mashed, with 2 tablespoons chunky salsa and 2 tablespoons fat-free sour cream

22 baked tortilla chips

Daily totals: 1,785 calories, 42 g total fat, 8.3 g saturated fat, 86 mg cholesterol, 25 g dietary fiber, 2,496 mg sodium

Day 24

Breakfast

1 cup oatmeal with 1 tablespoon brown sugar and ½ cup fat-free milk

1 tangerine or other seasonal fruit

Lunch

1 cup low-sodium black bean soup

1 cup polenta with 1 cup stewed tomatoes (with onions) and ⅛ teaspoon ground chile pepper

½ cup grapes

Dinner

Tossed salad: 2 cups chopped romaine lettuce, ¼ cup frozen or canned plain artichoke hearts, and ¼ sweet red pepper, chopped, dressed with 2 teaspoons olive oil and 2 tablespoons vinegar

3 ounces roasted skinless chicken breast

Three-grain pilaf: ⅓ cup steamed rice, ⅓ cup steamed barley, and ⅓ cup steamed buckwheat, tossed with ¼ cup diced onions, ¼ cup diced celery, and ¼ cup diced mushrooms sautéed in chicken stock, ¼ teaspoon dried tarragon, ¼ teaspoon rosemary, and ¼ teaspoon dry mustard

1 cup steamed sliced carrots and beets, dressed with 2 teaspoons olive oil, 2 teaspoons vinegar, and ½ teaspoon basil

Snack

2 rye crackers with 1 ounce low-fat mozzarella cheese

Daily totals: 2,201 calories, 38 g total fat, 8.9 g saturated fat, 78 mg cholesterol, 22 g dietary fiber, 1,485 mg sodium

Day 25

Breakfast

1 slice toasted whole wheat bread with 2 teaspoons diet margarine

½ cup fat-free vanilla yogurt with 2 chopped dried figs and 2 teaspoons wheat germ

Lunch

Chef's salad: 2 cups chopped mixed greens (romaine lettuce and spinach) with 1 ounce shredded fat-free Swiss cheese, 1 ounce julienne roasted turkey (without skin), ¼ cup sliced cucumbers, ¼ cup sliced radishes, ½ cup shredded carrots, and 3 or 4 cherry tomatoes, dressed with 2 tablespoons fat-free dressing (your choice)

3 breadsticks (1¼ ounces each)

1 cup unsweetened applesauce with cinnamon

Dinner

3 ounces broiled salmon

1½ cups white and wild rice with 2 teaspoons slivered almonds, 1 tablespoon sautéed diced onions, 2 teaspoons chopped parsley, and a pinch of saffron

1 artichoke, dressed with 1 tablespoon lemon juice, 1 teaspoon olive oil, 1 tablespoon fat-free Parmesan cheese, and butter-flavored sprinkles

¼ wedge cantaloupe

Snack

Tropical shake: ½ cup fat-free milk, ½ cup orange juice, 1 banana, and 5 strawberries, whipped until thick and frothy

Daily totals: 1,734 calories, 32 g total fat, 6.9 g saturated fat, 80 mg cholesterol, 34 g dietary fiber, 2,089 mg sodium

Day 26

Breakfast

¾ cup ready-to-eat raisin bran cereal with ½ cup fat-free milk

1 peach

Lunch

1½ cups low-sodium turkey noodle soup

1 sweet potato, baked with 1 tablespoon maple syrup, cinnamon, and nutmeg

Spinach salad: 1 cup chopped spinach, ½ cup shredded carrots, ¼ cup alfalfa sprouts, and ¼ cup sliced onions, dressed with 2 teaspoons olive oil and 2 tablespoons vinegar

1 pumpernickel roll (1 ounce) with 1 teaspoon diet margarine

Mixed fruit: ½ cup canned unsweetened pears, ¼ cup sliced apples, ¼ cup grapes, 1 dried fig, 2 tablespoons raisins

Dinner

Vegetable lasagna (low-fat, low-calorie frozen entrée)

½ cup steamed sliced carrots with a dash of fresh or dried ginger

Garlic bread: 2 slices toasted Italian bread, brushed with 2 teaspoons olive oil and rubbed with 1 clove fresh garlic

1 lemon sorbet bar

Snacks

Tropical delight: ½ cup orange juice, 1 banana, sliced, and 1 tablespoon slivered almonds, whipped until frothy

2 popcorn rice cakes

Daily totals: 1,874 calories, 39 g total fat, 4.7 g saturated fat, 29 mg cholesterol, 32 g dietary fiber, 2,215 mg sodium

Day 27

Breakfast

Two 4-inch whole grain pancakes

Scrambled eggs: ¼ cup egg substitute, scrambled with 1 tablespoon fat-free milk in a nonstick pan

1 ounce turkey sausage

Lunch

Rice jambalaya: 1½ cups cooked rice with ¼ cup cooked diced ham, ¼ cup cooked cubed chicken breast, ¼ cup crushed tomatoes, ¼ cup diced celery, ¼ cup chopped onions, ¼ cup chopped green peppers, and ¼ cup chopped mushrooms

2 buttermilk biscuits (¾ ounce each)

Fruit compote: 1 orange, sectioned, and 1 kiwifruit, sliced

Dinner

Stuffed potato: 1 baked potato with 2 ounces low-fat Cheddar cheese, ½ cup steamed broccoli, ¼ cup chopped onions, and 1 clove fresh garlic, minced

1 carrot, cut into sticks, with 1 tablespoon fat-free blue cheese dressing

½ cup fat-free pudding, made with fat-free milk

Snacks

1 bake-and-eat soft pretzel (2½ ounces, baked without salt)

1 stewed apple, topped with ¼ cup fat-free vanilla yogurt and drizzled with honey

Daily totals: 1,727 calories, 26 g total fat, 11 g saturated fat, 147 mg cholesterol, 24 g dietary fiber, 2,401 mg sodium

Day 28

Breakfast
1 toasted bagel with 2 tablespoons fat-free cream cheese and 1 tablespoon strawberry spread

1 cup vanilla fat-free yogurt

½ cup mixed berries

Lunch
3 ounces London broil (top round), marinated in ¼ teaspoon Worcestershire sauce, garlic, and herbs and grilled

2 ears grilled corn on the cob with butter-flavored sprinkles

Veggie kebabs: ½ cup chunked mushrooms, ½ cup chunked onions, and ½ cup chunked peppers, grilled on skewers and brushed with fat-free dressing (your choice)

2 breadsticks

2 cups cubed watermelon

Dinner
Pita pizza: 1 pita, smothered with ¼ cup tomato puree, 2 ounces shredded fat-free or reduced-fat mozzarella cheese, ⅓ cup sliced mushrooms, 1 clove fresh garlic, minced, and ¼ cup chopped onions

Tossed salad: 3 cups chopped greens, dressed with 2 tablespoons vinegar and 2 teaspoons olive oil

1 frozen fruit bar

Snack
2 cups air-popped popcorn with butter-flavored sprinkles

Daily totals: 1,735 calories, 38 g total fat, 14 g saturated fat, 121 mg cholesterol, 29 g dietary fiber, 1,707 mg sodium

Day 29

Breakfast

1 cup ready-to-eat oat cereal with almonds, topped with 1 banana, sliced, and ½ cup fat-free milk

½ grapefruit

Lunch

1 cup low-sodium chicken noodle soup

Ham and cheese sandwich: 1 ounce low-fat ham and 1 ounce low-fat American cheese on a hard roll (1 ounce) with lettuce, tomato, and mustard

1 carrot and 1 stalk celery, cut into sticks

Flavored sparkling water

Dinner

Turkey tenders: 3 ounces white-meat turkey, sautéed with 2 teaspoons olive oil, ½ cup chopped kale, ¼ cup sliced mushrooms, ¼ cup chopped onions, ¼ cup sliced bell peppers, and ¼ cup chopped hot peppers and served over 1 baked potato

Pasta salad: 1 cup cooked macaroni, ¼ cup chopped zucchini, ¼ cup chopped onions, and ¼ cup frozen or canned plain artichoke hearts, dressed with 2 tablespoons low-fat mayonnaise and sprinkled with basil and pepper

2 slices whole wheat bread with 2 teaspoons diet margarine

Snacks

1 apple

½ cup fat-free vanilla yogurt with 1 tablespoon chopped walnut topping

1 bake-and-eat soft pretzel (2½ ounces, baked without salt)

Daily totals: 1,959 calories, 42 g total fat, 5 g saturated fat, 57 mg cholesterol, 28 g dietary fiber, 2,020 mg sodium

Day 30

Breakfast

2 slices toasted raisin bread with $\frac{1}{2}$ cup reduced-fat ricotta cheese

1 banana

Lunch

1 cup low-sodium vegetarian chili, served over $1\frac{1}{2}$ cups steamed rice

Carrot and raisin salad: $\frac{1}{4}$ cup shredded carrots and $\frac{1}{4}$ cup raisins, served on $\frac{1}{2}$ cup chopped romaine lettuce with 2 tablespoons walnuts and dressed with 2 tablespoons fat-free yogurt and 1 tablespoon light mayonnaise

$\frac{1}{2}$ cup low-fat yogurt (your choice) with $\frac{1}{2}$ cup raspberries

Dinner

1 cup pasta

Red clam sauce: $\frac{1}{4}$ cup low-sodium stewed tomatoes, $\frac{1}{4}$ cup low-sodium tomato sauce, $\frac{1}{4}$ cup shredded carrots, and $1\frac{1}{2}$ ounces rinsed and chopped canned clams

1 slice Italian bread

2 almond biscotti or 1 fat-free cookie (your choice)

Snacks

4 small gingersnap cookies (1 ounce total)

1 pear

Daily totals: 2,103 calories, 37 g total fat, 10.5 g saturated fat, 76 mg cholesterol, 28 g dietary fiber, 1,182 mg sodium

PART THREE

The 500-Food Fat and Cholesterol Counter

Choose Foods That Work in Your Favor

Put away your calculator: The chart that begins on page 228 makes it easy to stick to a cholesterol-lowering diet. The best part? No number crunching is necessary (unless you want to do it, of course).

Like most other fat and cholesterol counters, this chart divvies up food into categories, from beans to vegetables. The key difference? It ranks foods by the amount of saturated fat per serving—"low," "acceptable," or "high"—rather than by the amount of dietary cholesterol. Most experts agree that saturated fat is the healthy heart's worst enemy. The more you stick to foods in the "low" category, the less saturated fat you'll eat and the healthier your diet will be.

As long as your overall calorie and cholesterol intake is reasonable, that is. Some foods contain a low percentage of saturated fat but pack lots of calories and cholesterol. For example, both 3 ounces of tofu and a fast-food ham-and-cheese breakfast croissant get 54 percent of their calories from fat. But compare the calories, cholesterol, and saturated fat content, and it's easy to see why breakfast croissants should be an occasional indulgence.

Here's some other information that you'll need to use this chart.

• We've rounded calorie and cholesterol counts to the nearest whole number and fat and saturated fat values to the nearest tenth of a gram.

• Foods that get less than 1 percent of their calories per serving from fat or saturated fat are designated by "<1."

• Unless otherwise specified, the foods are commercially prepared.

• While brand names are used in some cases, the nutrient information for many commercially prepared foods should be viewed as sample values. Expect variations among different brands and read labels carefully.

• Since beans, fruits, and vegetables typically contain little or no saturated fat and cholesterol, we've devoted the most space to other food categories.

Food	Portion	Calories	Fat (g)
Beans, Bean Products, and Other Legumes			
LOW			
Adzuki beans, boiled	½ cup	147	0.1
Baked beans with pork, canned	½ cup	134	2
Black beans, boiled	½ cup	114	0.5
Broad beans (fava beans), boiled	½ cup	94	0.3
Chickpeas, canned	½ cup	143	1.4
Green peas, boiled	½ cup	67	0.2
Lentils, boiled	½ cup	114	0.4
Lima beans, boiled	½ cup	108	0.4
Refried beans, canned	½ cup	135	1.4
Snap beans (green beans), boiled	½ cup	22	0.2
Soybeans, boiled	½ cup	149	7.7
Soybean sprouts, raw	½ cup	45	2.4
Split peas, boiled	½ cup	116	0.4
Three-bean salad, canned	⅓ cup	100	0.5
Tempeh	½ cup	165	6.4
ACCEPTABLE			
Tofu, firm, raw	¼ block (about 3 oz)	118	7.1
HIGH			
Chili, vegetarian, canned	1 cup	286	14
Chili with beans and meat, canned	1 cup	250	11
Breads and Bread Products			
LOW			
Bagel, plain or onion	1 (about 2½ oz)	195	1.1
Blueberry muffin			
homemade with 2% milk	1 (about 2 oz)	163	6.2
low-fat, frozen	1 (about 2½ oz)	190	5
Breadstick, plain	1 (about ¼ oz)	25	0.6
Cornbread, homemade with 2% milk	1 piece (about 2¼ oz)	173	4.6

Saturated Fat (g)	% Calories from Fat	% Calories from Saturated Fat	Cholesterol (mg)
0	<1	<1	0
0.8	13.4	5.4	9
0.1	3.9	<1	0
0.1	2.9	1	0
0.1	8.8	<1	0
0.1	2.7	<1	0
0.1	3.2	<1	0
0.1	3.3	<1	0
0.5	9.3	3.3	0
0	8.2	1.6	0
1.1	46.5	6.6	0
0.3	48	6	0
0.1	3.1	<1	0
0	4.5	0	0
0.9	34.9	4.9	0
1	54.1	7.6	0
6	44.1	18.9	43
5	39.6	18	50
0.2	5.1	<1	0
1.2	34.2	6.6	21
1	23.7	4.7	5
0.1	21.6	3.6	0
1	23.9	5.2	26

(continued)

Food	Portion	Calories	Fat (g)
Breads and Bread Products *(cont.)*			
LOW *(cont.)*			
Corn muffin, homemade with 2% milk	1 (about 2 oz)	180	7
Cracked wheat bread	1 slice (about 1 oz)	65	1
English muffin, plain, toasted	1 (about 2 oz)	133	1
French, Vienna, or sourdough bread	1 slice (about 1 oz)	69	0.8
Italian bread	1 slice (about 1 oz)	81	1.1
Pita, white	1 (about 2 oz)	165	0.7
Pumpernickel bread	1 slice (about 1 oz)	80	1
Raisin bread	1 slice (about 1 oz)	71	1.1
Roll or bun, homemade with whole milk	1 (about 1 oz)	112	2.7
Rye bread	1 slice (about 1 oz)	83	1.1
Wheat bread, reduced-calorie	1 slice (about 1 oz)	46	0.5
White bread, soft crumb	1 slice (about 1 oz)	67	0.9
ACCEPTABLE			
Biscuit, buttermilk, refrigerator	2 (about 2 oz total)	170	7
Bran muffin, homemade with wheat bran and 2% milk	1 (about 2 oz)	161	7
Cinnamon roll, refrigerator, baked, with frosting	1 (about 1 oz)	109	4
Zwieback rusks	5 pieces (about 1 oz)	149	3.4
HIGH			
Biscuit, baking powder, homemade	1 (about 1 oz)	103	4.8
Croissant	1 (about 2 oz)	235	12
Popover, homemade	1 (about 1½ oz)	90	3.7
Spoon bread, homemade with vegetable shortening	1 slice	468	27.4
Breakfast Foods			
LOW			
Danish, cinnamon nut (Arby's)	1 (3½ oz)	360	11
French toast, frozen, with low-calorie syrup	2 slices (about 4 oz total) with 4 Tbsp syrup	340	6

Saturated Fat (g)	% Calories from Fat	% Calories from Saturated Fat	Cholesterol (mg)
1.3	35	6.5	24
0.2	13.8	2.8	0
0.2	6.8	1.4	0
0.2	10.4	2.6	0
0.3	12.2	3.3	0
0.1	3.8	<1	0
0.1	11.3	1.1	0
0.3	13.9	3.8	0
0.7	21.7	5.6	13
0.2	11.9	2.2	0
0.1	9.8	2	0
0.2	12.1	2.7	<1
1.5	37.1	7.9	0
1.3	39.1	7.3	19
1	33	8.3	0
1.4	20.5	8.3	7
1.2	41.9	10.5	1
3.5	46	13.4	13
1.3	37	13	59
8.7	52.7	16.7	293
1	27.5	2.5	0
1.5	15.9	4	80

(continued)

Food	Portion	Calories	Fat (g)
Breakfast Foods *(cont.)*			
LOW *(cont.)*			
Hash browns, frozen, oven-heated	1 patty (about 2½ oz)	110	6
Pancakes with 2 pats butter and syrup (McDonald's)	3 (about 9 oz total)	560	14
Toaster pastry with fruit	1	204	5.3
Waffle, frozen, with low-calorie syrup	1 (about 1¼ oz) with 2 Tbsp syrup	136	2.1
ACCEPTABLE			
Coffee cake, caramel nut	1 slice (about 2 oz)	240	12
Doughnut, plain, made without yeast	1 (about 2 oz)	198	10.8
HIGH			
Biscuit with egg, cheese, and sausage, frozen	1 (about 5½ oz)	490	30
Biscuit with egg and sausage (McDonald's)	1 (about 6½ oz)	520	35
Croissant with egg, cheese, and sausage (Burger King)	1 (about 6 oz)	530	41
Croissant with ham and cheese (Arby's)	1 (about 4¼ oz)	345	20.7
Danish, cheese (McDonald's)	1 (about 4 oz)	410	22
Doughnut, cream-filled, yeast or raised	1 (about 3 oz)	307	20.8
English muffin with egg, cheese, and Canadian bacon (McDonald's)	1 (about 5 oz)	290	13
French toast sticks without butter and syrup (Burger King)	5 (about 5½ oz total)	500	27
Hash browns (McDonald's)	1 patty (about 2 oz)	130	8
Cold Cereals			
LOW			
Cheerios with fat-free milk	1 cup with ½ cup milk	150	2
Granola without raisins, low-fat, with fat-free milk	1 cup with ½ cup milk	250	3

Saturated Fat (g)	% Calories from Fat	% Calories from Saturated Fat	Cholesterol (mg)
0	49.1	0	0
2.5	22.5	4	10
0.8	23.4	3.5	0
0.5	13.9	3.3	0
2.5	45	9.4	20
1.8	49.1	8.2	17
12	55.1	22	145
10	60.6	17.3	245
14	69.6	23.8	255
12.1	54	31.6	90
8	48.3	17.6	70
5.7	61	16.7	20
4.5	40.3	14	235
7	48.6	12.6	0
1.5	55.4	10.4	0
0.5	12	3	<5
0	10.8	0	0

(continued)

Food	Portion	Calories	Fat (g)
Breakfast Foods *(cont.)*			
Cold Cereals *(cont.)*			
LOW *(cont.)*			
Kellogg's Frosted Flakes with fat-free milk	³/₄ cup with ¹/₂ cup milk	160	0
Raisin Bran with fat-free milk	1 cup with ¹/₂ cup milk	210	1
Shredded Wheat without milk	2 biscuits	160	0.5
Trix with fat-free milk	1 cup with ¹/₂ cup milk	160	1.5
ACCEPTABLE			
Cinnamon Toast Crunch with 2% milk	³/₄ cup with ¹/₂ cup milk	190	6
HIGH			
Cracklin' Oat Bran with fat-free milk	³/₄ cup with ¹/₂ cup milk	270	8
100% Natural with fruit and nuts, with 2% milk	²/₃ cup with ¹/₂ cup milk	310	13.5
Hot Cereals			
LOW			
Cream of Rice, cooked	³/₄ cup	95	0.2
Cream of Wheat, quick-cooking, cooked	³/₄ cup	97	0.4
Farina, enriched, cooked	³/₄ cup	88	0.2
Oatmeal, cooked	³/₄ cup	109	1.8
Ralston, cooked	³/₄ cup	101	0.6
Wheatena, cooked	³/₄ cup	102	0.9
Candy and Sweets			
LOW			
Butterscotch	4 pieces (about 1 oz total)	112	1
Hard candy	3 pieces (about ¹/₂ oz total)	60	0

Saturated Fat (g)	% Calories from Fat	% Calories from Saturated Fat	Cholesterol (mg)
0	0	0	0
0	4.3	0	0
0	2.8	0	0
0.5	8.4	2.8	<5
2	28.4	9.5	0
3	26.7	10	0
3.5	39.2	10.2	0
0	1.9	0	0
0	3.7	0	0
0	2	<1	0
0.3	14.9	2.5	0
0	5.3	0	0
0	7.9	0	0
0.3	8	2.4	3
0	0	0	0

(continued)

Food	Portion	Calories	Fat (g)
Candy and Sweets *(cont.)*			
LOW *(cont.)*			
Marshmallow chicks	5 small (about 2 oz total)	160	0
Peanut brittle	1 piece (about 1⅓ oz)	180	5
ACCEPTABLE			
Fudge, vanilla, homemade	1 piece (about 1 oz)	105	1.5
HIGH			
Almonds, chocolate-coated	7 (about 1 oz total)	159	12.2
Caramels	3 (about 1 oz total)	108	2.3
Chocolate bar, semisweet	1 (about 1½ oz)	230	13
Coconut bar, chocolate-coated	1 (about 2 oz)	195	11.7
Fudge, chocolate with nuts, homemade	1 piece (about 1 oz)	121	4.6
Mints, chocolate-coated	2 (about ⅓ oz total)	29	1.1
Peanuts, chocolate-coated	10 (about 1½ oz total)	208	13.4
Raisins, chocolate-coated	10 (about ⅓ oz total)	39	1.5
Vanilla creams, chocolate-coated	1 oz	122	4.8
Cheese and Cheese Products			
LOW			
American, fat-free	1 slice (about ¾ oz)	30	0
Cheddar, fat-free	1 oz	45	0
Cream cheese, fat-free	2 Tbsp	30	0
Swiss, fat-free	1 slice (about ¾ oz)	30	0
Yogurt cheese, low-fat	1 oz	30	0.6
ACCEPTABLE			
Cottage cheese, 1%	½ cup	82	1.2

Saturated Fat (g)	% Calories from Fat	% Calories from Saturated Fat	Cholesterol (mg)
0	0	0	0
1	25	5	0
1	12.9	8.6	5
2.1	69.1	11.9	0
1.9	19.2	15.8	2
9	50.9	35.2	10
6.2	54	28.6	0
1.6	34.2	11.9	4
0.7	34.1	21.7	0
5.8	58	25.1	4
0.9	34.6	20.8	1
1.4	35.4	10.3	1
0	0	0	0
0	0	0	25
0	0	0	5
0	0	0	0
Trace	18	Trace	0
0.7	13.2	7.7	5

(continued)

Food	Portion	Calories	Fat (g)
Cheese and Cheese Products *(cont.)*			
HIGH			
American	1 oz	106	8.9
Blue cheese	1 oz	99	8.1
Brie	1 oz	93	7.6
Camembert	1 oz	84	6.8
Caraway	1 oz	105	8.2
Cheddar			
reduced-fat	1 oz	80	5
regular	1 oz	110	9
Colby	1 oz	110	9
Cottage cheese			
creamed, small or large curd	½ cup	109	4.7
2%	½ cup	101	2.2
Cream cheese			
reduced-fat	2 Tbsp	70	5
regular	1 oz	100	10
Feta	1 oz	74	6
Fondue	¼ cup	151	10.4
Gouda	1 oz	100	7.7
Gruyère	1 oz	116	9.1
Limburger	1 oz	92	7.6
Monterey Jack	1 oz	105	8.5
Mozzarella			
reduced-fat	1 oz	71	4.5
regular	1 oz	79	6.1
Muenster			
reduced-fat	1 oz	80	5
regular	1 oz	103	8.4
Neufchâtel	1 oz	73	6.6
Parmesan, grated	1 Tbsp	23	1.5
Provolone	1 oz	98	7.5

Saturated Fat (g)	% Calories from Fat	% Calories from Saturated Fat	Cholesterol (mg)
5.6	75.6	47.5	27
5.2	73.6	47.3	21
4.9	73.5	47.4	28
4.3	72.9	46.1	20
5.2	70.3	44.6	26
3	56.3	33.8	20
6	73.6	49	30
5.7	73.6	46.6	27
3	38.8	24.8	16
1.4	19.6	12.5	10
3.5	64.3	45	15
6	90	54	30
4.2	72.9	51.1	25
5.1	62	30.4	128
4.9	69.3	44.1	32
5.3	70.6	41.1	31
4.7	74.3	46	25
5.3	72.9	45.4	25
2.8	57	35.5	16
3.7	69.5	42.2	22
3	56.3	33.8	20
5.4	73.4	47.2	27
4.1	81.4	50.5	21
1	58.7	39.1	4
4.8	68.9	44.1	19

(continued)

Food	Portion	Calories	Fat (g)
Cheese and Cheese Products *(cont.)*			

HIGH *(cont.)*

Food	Portion	Calories	Fat (g)
Ricotta			
reduced-fat	½ cup	171	9.8
regular	½ cup	216	16.1
Romano, grated	1 Tbsp	19	1.4
Soufflé, homemade	1 cup	207	16.2
Swiss	1 oz	105	7.7
Welsh rarebit, frozen	¼ cup (about 2 oz)	120	9

Desserts			
Cakes			

LOW

Food	Portion	Calories	Fat (g)
Angel food	1 slice (¹⁄₁₂ of cake)	73	0.2
Fruitcake	1 slice (about 2 oz)	139	3.9
Sponge	1 slice (¹⁄₁₂ of cake)	110	1

ACCEPTABLE

Food	Portion	Calories	Fat (g)
Boston cream	1 slice (⅙ of cake)	232	7.8
Devil's food, made from mix with eggs and oil, with 2 Tbsp chocolate icing	1 slice (¹⁄₁₂ of cake)	440	21
Pound, made with margarine	1 slice (¹⁄₁₆ of loaf cake)	206	9
White, made from mix with egg whites and oil, with 2 Tbsp reduced-calorie chocolate icing	1 slice (¹⁄₁₂ of cake)	370	11

HIGH

Food	Portion	Calories	Fat (g)
Carrot cake, homemade with cream cheese icing	1 slice (¹⁄₁₂ of cake)	484	29.3
Cheesecake, frozen	¼ cake (about 4¼ oz)	350	18
Pound, made with butter	1 slice (¹⁄₁₂ of cake)	110	5.6
Yellow with pudding, made from mix with eggs and margarine, with 2 Tbsp chocolate icing	1 slice (¹⁄₁₂ of cake)	410	17

Saturated Fat (g)	% Calories from Fat	% Calories from Saturated Fat	Cholesterol (mg)
6.1	51.6	32.1	38
10.3	67.1	42.9	63
0.9	66.3	42.6	5
8.2	70.4	35.7	176
5	66	42.9	26
4	67.5	30	20
0	2.5	<1	0
0.5	25.3	3.2	2
0.3	8.2	2.5	39
2.3	30.3	8.9	35
4.5	43	9.2	45
1.9	39.3	8.3	41
3	26.8	7.3	0
5.4	54.5	10	60
9	46.3	23.1	50
3.2	45.8	26.2	63
7.5	37.3	16.5	75

(continued)

Food	Portion	Calories	Fat (g)
Desserts *(cont.)*			
Cookies			
LOW			
Brownie with nuts, made from mix	1 (about ³/₄ oz)	81	3.7
Fig bars, fat-free	2 (about 1 oz total)	100	0
Gingersnaps	5 (about 1¼ oz total)	147	3.1
Ladyfingers	4 (about 1½ oz total)	158	3.4
Molasses	2 (about 2 oz total)	274	6.9
Oatmeal with raisins			
homemade	1 (about ½ oz)	65	2.4
reduced-fat	2 (about 1 oz total)	110	2.5
ACCEPTABLE			
Fig bars	2 (about 1 oz total)	110	2.5
Peanut butter, homemade	1 (about ³/₄ oz)	95	4.8
Sugar, homemade with margarine	1 (about ½ oz)	66	3.3
HIGH			
Chocolate chip, homemade with margarine	1 (about ½ oz)	78	4.5
Macaroon, homemade	1 (about 1 oz)	97	3.1
Sandwich, vanilla with cream filling	4 (about 2 oz total)	297	13.5
Sugar wafer with cream filling	1 small	18	0.9
Vanilla wafers	8 (about 1 oz total)	150	7
Pies			
LOW			
Apple, low-fat, frozen	1 slice (⅕ of pie)	220	5
Pecan, fresh	1 slice (⅛ of pie)	431	23.6

Saturated Fat (g)	% Calories from Fat	% Calories from Saturated Fat	Cholesterol (mg)
0.6	41.1	6.6	13
0	0	0	0
0.8	19	4.9	14
1.1	19.4	6.7	157
1.7	22.7	5.6	25
0.5	33.2	6.9	5
0	20.5	0	0
1	20.5	8.2	0
0.9	45.5	8.5	6
0.7	45	9.5	4
1.3	51.9	15	5
2.7	28.8	25.1	0
3.7	41	11.2	23
0.2	45	10	0
2	42	12	0
1	20.5	4.1	0
3.3	49.3	6.9	65

(continued)

Food	Portion	Calories	Fat (g)
Desserts *(cont.)*			
Pies *(cont.)*			
ACCEPTABLE			
Rhubarb, fresh	1 slice (1/8 of pie)	299	12.6
HIGH			
Apple, fresh	1 slice (1/8 of pie)	302	13.1
Banana custard, fresh	1 slice (1/8 of pie)	252	10.6
Blueberry, fresh	1 slice (1/8 of pie)	286	12.7
Cherry, fresh	1 slice (1/8 of pie)	308	13.3
Chocolate meringue, fresh	1 slice (1/8 of pie)	287	13.7
Custard, fresh	1 slice (1/8 of pie)	249	12.7
Lemon meringue, fresh	1 slice (1/8 of pie)	268	10.7
Mince, fresh	1 slice (1/8 of pie)	320	13.6
Pumpkin, fresh	1 slice (1/8 of pie)	241	12.8
Pudding			
ACCEPTABLE			
Vanilla, made from mix with 2% milk	1/2 cup	148	2.4
HIGH			
Chocolate, made from mix with whole milk	1/2 cup	163	4.6
Custard, homemade, baked	1/2 cup	148	6.6
Rice with raisins, homemade	1/2 cup	194	4.1
Tapioca, made from mix with whole milk	1/2 cup	161	4.1
Other			
LOW			
Fruit cocktail, canned in light syrup	1/2 cup	72	0.1
Gelatin, made from powder, with fruit	1/2 cup	80	0.1
HIGH			
Coconut cream, canned	1/2 cup	142	13.1
Eclair	1 (about 3 1/2 oz)	239	13.6

Saturated Fat (g)	% Calories from Fat	% Calories from Saturated Fat	Cholesterol (mg)
3.1	37.9	9.3	0
3.4	39	10.1	0
3.4	37.9	12.1	66
3.2	40	10.1	0
3.5	38.9	10.2	0
5.1	43	16	64
4.3	45.9	15.5	120
3.2	35.9	10.7	98
3.6	38.3	10.1	1
4.5	47.8	16.8	70
1.4	14.6	8.5	9
2.7	25.4	14.9	16
3.3	40.1	20.1	123
2.2	19	10.2	15
2.5	22.9	14	17
0	1.3	<1	0
0	1.1	0	0
11.6	83	73.5	0
4.4	51.2	16.6	136

(continued)

Food	Portion	Calories	Fat (g)
Dips and Snacks			
Dips			
LOW			
Hummus	1/3 cup	140	6.9
Onion, low-fat	2 Tbsp	30	0
Salsa	2 Tbsp	10	0
HIGH			
Bacon and horseradish	2 Tbsp	60	5
Cheese			
low-fat	2 Tbsp	80	3
regular	2 Tbsp	90	7
Clam	2 Tbsp	50	4.5
Onion	2 Tbsp	60	5
Ranch	2 Tbsp	140	14
Snacks			
LOW			
Caramel corn	1/2 cup	140	4
Cereal mix	3/4 cup	130	5
Cracker Jacks	1 box	150	3
Crackers			
graham	1 (1/2 oz)	55	1.3
saltines	5 (1/2 oz total)	61	1.7
Crispbread, rye	1 slice	35	0
Fruit rolls	2	110	1
Granola bar, chocolate chip, low-fat	1 (about 1 oz)	110	2
Melba toast	3 pieces (about 1/2 oz total)	55	0.5
Popcorn			
air-popped, plain	1 cup	31	0.3
microwave, butter-flavored, light	1 bag (about 13 cups)	110	4
Potato chips, fat-free	30 (about 1 oz total)	110	0

Saturated Fat (g)	% Calories from Fat	% Calories from Saturated Fat	Cholesterol (mg)
1	44.4	6.4	0
0	0	0	<5
0	0	0	0
3	75	45	20
2	33.6	22.5	15
5	70	50	20
3	81	54	20
3	75	45	20
2.5	90	16.1	10
1	25.7	6.4	<5
1	34.6	6.9	0
0.5	18	3	0
0.3	21.3	4.9	0
0.4	25.1	5.9	0
0	0	0	0
Trace	8.2	Trace	0
0.5	16.4	4.1	0
0.1	8.2	1.6	0
0.1	8.7	2.9	0
0.5	32.7	4.1	0
0	0	0	0

(continued)

Food	Portion	Calories	Fat (g)
Dips and Snacks *(cont.)*			
Snacks *(cont.)*			
LOW *(cont.)*			
Pretzels			
baked	16 (about 1 oz total)	120	2.5
cheese-flavored	1 oz	160	7
Dutch-type	2 large (about 1 oz total)	125	1.4
Rice cakes, flavored	1 (about $\frac{1}{2}$ oz)	50	0
Toffee corn (popcorn and peanuts)	$\frac{2}{3}$ cup (about 1 oz)	140	4
Tortilla chips, plain	13 (about 1 oz total)	140	6
ACCEPTABLE			
Corn chips	30 small (about 1 oz total)	155	9.1
Popcorn, microwave			
butter-flavored	1 bag (about 13 cups)	150	10
plain	1 bag (about 13 cups)	140	10
HIGH			
Cheez Doodles	17 (about 1 oz total)	150	8
Crackers			
butter-flavored	4 (about $\frac{1}{2}$ oz total)	64	2.5
cheese	4 round ($\frac{1}{2}$ oz total)	67	3
cheese and peanut butter	2 ($\frac{1}{2}$ oz total)	69	3.4
wheat	7 ($\frac{1}{2}$ oz total)	61	1.8
Granola bar, chocolate chip	1 (about 1 oz)	120	3.5
Popcorn, buttered	1 cup	41	2
Potato chips	10 (about $\frac{3}{4}$ oz total)	105	7.1
Potato sticks	1 oz	148	9.8
Sesame sticks	30 pieces (about 1 oz total)	170	12
Wheat Nuts (wheat germ nuggets)	1 oz	200	19

Saturated Fat (g)	% Calories from Fat	% Calories from Saturated Fat	Cholesterol (mg)
0	18.8	0	0
1	39.4	5.6	0
0.3	10.1	2.2	0
0	0	0	0
1	25.7	6.4	<5
1	38.6	6.4	0
1.5	52.8	8.7	0
1.5	60	9	0
1.5	64.3	9.6	0
2.5	48	15	0
0.8	35.2	11.3	0
1.2	40.2	16.1	4
0.9	44.3	11.7	2
0.9	26.6	13.3	0
1.5	26.3	11.3	0
0.9	43.9	19.8	4
1.8	60.9	15.4	0
2.5	59.6	15.2	0
2	63.5	10.6	0
3	85.5	13.5	0

(continued)

Food	Portion	Calories	Fat (g)
Dressings			
LOW			
Blue cheese, fat-free	2 Tbsp	35	0
Caesar, low-fat	2 Tbsp	70	6
French, fat-free	2 Tbsp	50	0
Garlic, creamy, fat-free	2 Tbsp	40	0
Honey Dijon, fat-free	2 Tbsp	50	0
Italian			
low-fat	2 Tbsp	15	0.5
fat-free	2 Tbsp	15	0
Oil and vinegar, imitation, fat-free	2 Tbsp	15	0
Ranch			
low-fat	2 Tbsp	80	7
fat-free	2 Tbsp	45	0
Thousand Island			
low-fat	2 Tbsp	45	1
fat-free	2 Tbsp	35	0
ACCEPTABLE			
French, low-fat	2 Tbsp	50	3
Ranch	2 Tbsp	140	14
Russian	2 Tbsp	110	6
HIGH			
Blue cheese			
low-fat	2 Tbsp	80	8
regular	2 Tbsp	170	17
Caesar	2 Tbsp	170	18
French	2 Tbsp	120	12
Garlic, creamy	2 Tbsp	140	13
Honey Dijon	2 Tbsp	130	10
Italian	2 Tbsp	100	10
Italian, creamy			
low-fat	2 Tbsp	50	5
regular	2 Tbsp	110	11

Saturated Fat (g)	% Calories from Fat	% Calories from Saturated Fat	Cholesterol (mg)
0	0	0	0
0.5	77.1	6.4	5
0	0	0	0
0	0	0	0
0	0	0	0
0	30	0	0
0	0	0	0
0	0	0	0
0.5	78.8	5.6	0
0	0	0	0
0	20	0	<5
0	0	0	0
0.5	54	9	0
1.5	90	9.6	10
1	49.1	8.2	0
2	90	22.5	0
3	90	15.9	10
2.5	95.3	13.2	0
2	90	15	0
2	83.6	12.9	0
1.5	69.2	10.4	0
1.5	90	13.5	0
1	90	18	0
4	90	32.7	0

(continued)

Food	Portion	Calories	Fat (g)
Dressings *(cont.)*			
HIGH *(cont.)*			
Oil and vinegar			
low-fat	2 Tbsp	60	5
regular	2 Tbsp	110	11
Sweet-and-sour	2 Tbsp	150	13
Thousand Island	2 Tbsp	110	10
Eggs and Egg Substitute			
LOW			
Egg white	1 large	16	Trace
ACCEPTABLE			
Egg substitute, liquid	¼ cup	53	2.1
HIGH			
Egg			
fried with margarine	1 large	92	6.9
hard-cooked	1 large	78	5.3
scrambled with butter and whole milk	1 large	95	7.1
Egg substitute, frozen	¼ cup	96	6.7
Egg yolk	1 large	59	5.1
Quiche			
Lorraine	1 slice (about 6¼ oz)	600	48
spinach, frozen	1 (about 6 oz)	480	32
Fast Foods			
LOW			
Baked potato with cheese and bacon (Wendy's)	1 (about 10 oz)	530	18
BBQ Beef sandwich on bun (Dairy Queen/Brazier)	1 (about 4 oz)	225	4
Fish, breaded, baked, without bun (Long John Silver's)	3 pieces (about 5 oz total)	150	1
Onion rings, breaded (Burger King)	1 order (about 5 oz)	310	14

Saturated Fat (g)	% Calories from Fat	% Calories from Saturated Fat	Cholesterol (mg)
1	75	15	0
2	90	16.4	0
2	78	12	0
1.5	81.8	12.3	10
0	Trace	0	0
0.4	35.7	7	1
1.9	67.5	18.6	211
1.6	61.2	18.5	212
2.8	67.3	26.5	248
1.2	62.8	11.3	1
1.6	77.8	24.4	213
23.2	72	34.8	285
16	60	30	205
4	30.6	6.8	20
1	16	4	20
0.6	6	3.6	110
2	40.6	5.8	0

(continued)

Food	Portion	Calories	Fat (g)
Fast Foods *(cont.)*			
ACCEPTABLE			
Baked potato with sour cream and chives (Wendy's)	1 (about 10 oz)	380	6
Burrito, bean (Taco Bell)	1	391	12
Chicken, breaded, with mayonnaise, lettuce, and tomato on bun (Wendy's)	1 (about 9 oz)	450	20
Chicken breast and wing quarter, roasted, without skin (KFC)	1 (about 4 oz total)	199	5.9
Fish, breaded, with tartar sauce on bun (McDonald's)	1 (about 6 oz)	360	16
French fries (McDonald's)	1 large (about 6 oz)	450	22
Garden salad with 2 Tbsp reduced-fat, reduced-calorie Italian dressing (Wendy's)	1 (about 10 oz)	150	9
Pie, apple (Burger King)	1 (about 4 oz)	310	15
Shake, chocolate (McDonald's)	1 small (about 16 oz)	350	6
HIGH			
Baked potato with chili and cheese (Wendy's)	1 (about 10 oz)	610	24
Baked potato with broccoli and cheese (Arby's)	1 (about 10 oz)	417	17.9
Burrito, chicken (Taco Bell)	1	345	13
Cheeseburger with condiments on bun (Burger King)	1 (about 5 oz)	320	13
Cheese steak with onions and peppers on bun (Arby's)	1 (about 7 oz)	467	25.3
Chef's salad with turkey, ham, cheese, and Thousand Island dressing (Arby's)	1 (about 14 oz)	503	38.7
Chicken breast, fried (KFC)	1 (about 5 oz)	360	20
Chicken nuggets without sauce (KFC)	6 (about 3 oz total)	284	18
Double cheeseburger with condiments on bun (Burger King)	1 (about 8 oz)	600	36
Hamburger with condiments on bun (McDonald's)	1 (about 4 oz)	270	9

Saturated Fat (g)	% Calories from Fat	% Calories from Saturated Fat	Cholesterol (mg)
4	14.2	9.5	15
4	27.6	9.2	5
4	40	8	60
1.7	26.7	7.7	97
3.5	40	8.8	35
4	44	8	0
1.5	54	9	0
3	43.5	8.7	0
3.5	15.4	9	25
9	35.4	13.3	45
6.9	38.6	14.9	22
5	33.9	13	57
6	36.6	16.9	40
9.7	48.8	18.7	53
8.2	69.2	14.7	150
5	50	12.5	115
4	57	12.7	68
17	54	25.5	135
3	30	10	30

(continued)

Food	Portion	Calories	Fat (g)
Fast Foods *(cont.)*			
HIGH *(cont.)*			
Hot dog, plain, on bun (Dairy Queen/ Brazier)	1 (about 3 oz)	280	16
Nachos Supreme (Taco Bell)	1 order	364	18
Roast beef on bun (Arby's)	1 (about 6 oz)	383	18.2
Shake, vanilla (McDonald's)	1 small (about 16 oz)	310	5
Submarine			
Italian (cold cuts) (Arby's)	1 (about 10 oz)	671	38.8
Tuna (Arby's)	1 (about 10 oz)	663	37
Taco, beef (Taco Bell)	1	180	11
Taco salad with small chili and 1 packet sour cream (Wendy's)	1 (about 30 oz)	830	42
Tostada (Taco Bell)	1	242	11
Fats, Oils, and Spreads			
Fats			
HIGH			
Chicken	1 Tbsp	115	12.8
Lard	1 Tbsp	115	12.8
Shortening	1 Tbsp	113	12.8
Oils			
ACCEPTABLE			
Almond	1 Tbsp	120	13.6
Canola	1 Tbsp	124	14
Grapeseed	1 Tbsp	120	13.6
Safflower	1 Tbsp	120	13.6
Walnut	1 Tbsp	120	13.6
HIGH			
Avocado	1 Tbsp	124	14
Coconut	1 Tbsp	120	13.6
Corn	1 Tbsp	120	13.6

Saturated Fat (g)	% Calories from Fat	% Calories from Saturated Fat	Cholesterol (mg)
6	51.4	19.3	25
5	44.5	12.4	17
7	42.8	16.4	43
3.5	14.5	10.2	25
12.8	52	17.2	69
8.2	50.2	11.1	43
5	55	25	32
17.5	45.5	19	125
4	40.9	14.9	14
3.8	100	29.7	11
5	100	39.1	4
3.2	100	25.5	0
1.1	100	8.3	0
1	100	7.3	0
1.3	100	9.8	0
1.2	100	9	0
1.2	100	9	0
1.6	100	11.6	0
11.8	100	88.5	0
1.7	100	12.8	0

(continued)

Food	Portion	Calories	Fat (g)
Fats, Oils, and Spreads *(cont.)*			
Oils *(cont.)*			
HIGH *(cont.)*			
Cottonseed	1 Tbsp	120	13.6
Olive	1 Tbsp	119	13.5
Palm	1 Tbsp	120	13.6
Peanut	1 Tbsp	119	13.5
Sesame	1 Tbsp	120	13.6
Soybean	1 Tbsp	120	13.6
Sunflower	1 Tbsp	120	13.6
Spreads			
LOW			
Apple butter	1 Tbsp	33	0.1
Mayonnaise, low-fat	1 Tbsp	25	1
ACCEPTABLE			
Almond butter, unsalted	1 Tbsp	101	9.5
Peanut butter without added oils	2 Tbsp	200	16
HIGH			
Butter, salted, unsalted stick, or whipped	1 Tbsp	102	11.5
Butter blend, made with butter and vegetable oil	1 Tbsp	50	6
Margarine			
squeeze	1 Tbsp	80	9
stick			
reduced-fat	1 Tbsp	60	6
regular	1 Tbsp	100	11
tub			
reduced-fat	1 Tbsp	45	4.5
regular	1 Tbsp	100	11
Mayonnaise			
reduced-fat	1 Tbsp	50	5
regular	1 Tbsp	100	11
Peanut butter with added oils, smooth	2 Tbsp	188	16

Saturated Fat (g)	% Calories from Fat	% Calories from Saturated Fat	Cholesterol (mg)
3.5	100	26.3	0
1.8	100	13.6	0
6.7	100	50.3	0
2.3	100	17.4	0
1.9	100	14.3	0
2	100	15	0
1.4	100	10.5	0
0	2.7	0	0
0	36	0	0
0.9	84.7	8	0
2	72	9	0
7.2	100	63.5	31
3	100	54	10
1.5	100	16.9	0
1	90	15	0
2	99	18	0
1	90	20	0
2	99	18	0
1	90	18	5
1.5	99	13.5	5
3.1	76.6	14.8	0

(continued)

Food	Portion	Calories	Fat (g)
Fish and Shellfish			
Fish			
LOW			
Bass, striped, uncooked	3 oz	82	2
Bluefish, uncooked	3 oz	105	3.6
Cod, Atlantic, broiled, baked, or microwaved	3 oz	89	0.7
Flounder, broiled, baked, or microwaved	3 oz	99	1.3
Grouper, broiled, baked, or microwaved	3 oz	100	1.1
Haddock, broiled, baked, or microwaved	3 oz	95	0.8
Halibut, broiled, baked, or microwaved	3 oz	119	2.5
Mahi mahi, uncooked	3 oz	72	0.6
Monkfish, uncooked	3 oz	65	1.3
Ocean perch, Atlantic, broiled, baked, or microwaved	3 oz	103	1.8
Orange roughy, broiled, baked, or microwaved	3 oz	75	0.8
Pollack, broiled, baked, or microwaved	3 oz	96	1
Shark, mixed species, uncooked	3 oz	111	3.8
Smelt, rainbow, broiled, baked, or microwaved	3 oz	105	2.6
Snapper, mixed species, broiled, baked, or microwaved	3 oz	109	1.5
Sole, broiled, baked, or microwaved	3 oz	99	1.3
Surimi, uncooked	3 oz	84	0.7
Trout, rainbow, broiled, baked, or microwaved	3 oz	128	3.7
Tuna, light meat, canned in water	3 oz	99	0.7
Turbot, European, uncooked	3 oz	81	2.5
Whitefish, mixed species, smoked	3 oz	92	0.8

Saturated Fat (g)	% Calories from Fat	% Calories from Saturated Fat	Cholesterol (mg)
0.4	22	4.4	68
0.8	30.9	6.9	50
0.1	7.1	1	47
0.3	11.8	2.7	58
0.3	9.9	2.7	40
0.1	7.6	<1	63
0.4	18.9	3	35
0.2	7.5	2.5	62
0.3	18	4.2	21
0.3	15.7	2.6	46
0	9.6	<1	22
0.2	9.4	1.9	82
0.8	30.8	6.5	43
0.5	22.3	4.3	77
0.3	12.4	2.5	40
0.3	11.8	2.7	58
0.2	7.5	2.1	26
0.7	26	4.9	62
0.2	6.4	1.8	26
0.6	27.8	6.7	41
0.2	7.8	2	28

(continued)

Food	Portion	Calories	Fat (g)
Fish and Shellfish *(cont.)*			
Fish *(cont.)*			
ACCEPTABLE			
Anchovies, canned in olive oil	5 (about ¾ oz total)	42	1.9
Carp, broiled, baked, or microwaved	3 oz	138	6.1
Salmon			
pink, canned, with bones and liquid	3 oz	118	5.1
sockeye, fresh, broiled, baked, or microwaved	3 oz	184	9.3
Sardines, Atlantic, canned in oil, drained, with bones	2 (about 1 oz total)	50	2.8
Swordfish, broiled, baked, or microwaved	3 oz	132	4.4
Tuna, fresh, broiled, baked, or microwaved	3 oz	156	5.3
Tuna salad, prepared with mayonnaise	3 oz	159	7.9
HIGH			
Catfish, channel, breaded and fried	3 oz	195	11.3
Caviar, black or red	1 Tbsp	40	2.9
Eel, broiled, baked, or microwaved	3 oz	201	12.7
Herring, kippered	1 fillet (about 1½ oz)	87	5
Mackerel, Atlantic, broiled, baked, or microwaved	3 oz	223	15.1
Pompano, Florida, broiled, baked, or microwaved	3 oz	179	10.3
Shellfish			
LOW			
Clams, steamed	20 small (about 3 oz)	133	1.8
Crab, Alaskan king, steamed	3 oz	82	1.3
Crayfish (crawfish), steamed	3 oz	97	1.2
Lobster, boiled, poached, or steamed	3 oz	83	0.5

Saturated Fat (g)	% Calories from Fat	% Calories from Saturated Fat	Cholesterol (mg)
0.4	40.7	8.6	17
1.2	39.8	7.8	71
1.3	38.9	9.9	47
1.6	45.5	7.8	74
0.4	50.4	7.2	34
1.2	30	8.2	43
1.4	30.6	8.1	42
1.3	44.7	7.4	11
2.8	52.2	12.9	69
0.7	65.3	15.6	94
2.6	56.9	11.6	137
1.1	51.7	11.4	33
3.6	60.9	14.5	64
3.8	51.8	19.1	54
0.2	12.2	1.4	60
0.1	14.3	1.1	45
0.2	11.1	1.9	151
0.1	5.4	1.1	61

(continued)

Food	Portion	Calories	Fat (g)
Fish and Shellfish *(cont.)*			
Shellfish *(cont.)*			
LOW *(cont.)*			
Mussels, blue, boiled, poached, or steamed	3 oz	146	3.8
Scallops, uncooked	3 oz	75	0.7
Shrimp, mixed species, steamed	3 oz	84	0.9
ACCEPTABLE			
Lobster salad, prepared with mayonnaise	½ cup	286	16.6
Oysters, eastern, steamed	6 medium (about 1½ oz total)	57	2.1
Shrimp, mixed species, breaded and fried	3 oz	206	10.4
HIGH			
Clams, mixed species, breaded and fried	20 small (about 6¾ oz total)	380	21
Crab, soft-shell, fried	1 (about 4½ oz)	334	17.9
Oysters, Eastern, breaded and fried	6 medium (about 3 oz total)	173	11.1
Scallops, mixed species, breaded and fried	2 large (about 1 oz total)	67	3.4
Fruits and Fruit Juices			
LOW			
Apple, raw, with skin	1 (about 5 oz)	81	0.5
Apple juice, unsweetened, canned or bottled	1 cup	117	0.3
Cherries, sweet, without pits	1 cup	104	1.4
Figs, dried	3 (about 2 oz total)	145	0.7
Grapefruit, pink	½ (about 4 oz)	37	0.1
Grapes, green or red	1 cup	114	0.9
Orange juice, frozen, from concentrate	1 cup	112	0.2
Peach, raw	1 (about 3 oz)	37	0.1
Pears, canned in light syrup	½ cup	72	0

Saturated Fat (g)	% Calories from Fat	% Calories from Saturated Fat	Cholesterol (mg)
0.7	23.4	4.3	48
0.1	8.4	1.2	28
0.3	9.8	3.2	166
2.6	52.2	8.2	120
0.6	33.2	9.5	44
1.8	45.4	7.9	151
5	49.7	11.8	115
4.4	48.2	11.9	45
2.8	57.7	14.6	71
0.8	45.7	10.7	19
0.1	5.5	1.1	0
0.1	2.3	<1	0
0.3	12.1	2.6	0
0.1	4.3	<1	0
0	2.4	<1	0
0.3	7.1	2.4	0
0	1.6	<1	0
0	2.4	<1	0
0	<1	0	0

(continued)

Food	Portion	Calories	Fat (g)
Fruits and Fruit Juices *(cont.)*			
LOW *(cont.)*			
Raisins, seedless	½ cup	218	0.3
Strawberries	1 cup	45	0.6
HIGH			
Avocado	½ (about 3 oz)	162	15.4
Grains			
LOW			
Barley, pearled, cooked	½ cup	97	0.4
Bran			
oat, raw	2 Tbsp	29	0.8
wheat, raw	2 Tbsp	15	0.3
Buckwheat groats, cooked	½ cup	91	0.6
Bulgur wheat, cooked	½ cup	76	0.2
Corn grits, white or yellow, cooked	½ cup	73	0.2
Cornmeal, whole grain, white or yellow, raw	¼ cup	109	1.1
Couscous, cooked	½ cup	101	0.1
Hominy, white or yellow, canned, raw	½ cup	58	0.7
Millet, cooked	½ cup	143	1.2
Quinoa, raw	¼ cup	159	2.5
Rye, raw	¼ cup	141	1.1
Wheat germ, toasted	¼ cup	108	3
HIGH			
Bran, rice, raw	2 Tbsp	33	2.2
Rice			
LOW			
Brown, cooked	½ cup	109	0.9
Chicken-flavored, made from mix with 2 Tbsp margarine (Rice-A-Roni)	1 cup	320	9.5
Fried, made from mix with 2 Tbsp margarine (Rice-A-Roni)	1 cup	320	11

Saturated Fat (g)	% Calories from Fat	% Calories from Saturated Fat	Cholesterol (mg)
0.1	1.2	<1	0
0	12	<1	0
2.5	85.6	13.9	0
0.1	3.7	<1	0
0.2	24.8	6.2	0
0	18	2.4	0
0.1	6	<1	0
0	2.4	<1	0
0	2.5	<1	0
0.2	9.1	1.7	0
0	<1	<1	0
0.1	10.9	1.6	0
0.2	7.5	1.3	0
0.3	14.2	1.7	0
0.1	7	<1	0
0.5	25	4.2	0
0.4	60	10.9	0
0.2	7.4	1.7	0
1	26.7	2.8	0
2	30.9	5.6	0

(continued)

Food	Portion	Calories	Fat (g)
Grains *(cont.)*			
Rice *(cont.)*			
LOW *(cont.)*			
Spanish, homemade	½ cup	107	2.1
White			
enriched, cooked	½ cup	133	0.3
instant, cooked	½ cup	80	0.1
Wild, cooked	½ cup	83	0.3
Gravies and Sauces			
Gravies			
LOW			
Mushroom, canned	¼ cup	30	1.6
Onion, dry mix, prepared	¼ cup	20	0.2
ACCEPTABLE			
Au jus, canned	¼ cup	10	0.1
Brown, dry mix, prepared	¼ cup	19	0.4
HIGH			
Beef, canned	¼ cup	31	1.4
Chicken, canned	¼ cup	47	3.4
Turkey, canned	¼ cup	30	1.3
Sauces			
LOW			
Barbecue, bottled	¼ cup	47	1.1
Marinara, canned	½ cup	85	4.2
Soy, tamari, bottled	1 Tbsp	11	0.1
Spaghetti, canned	½ cup	136	5.9
Sweet-and-sour, dry mix, made with water and vinegar	¼ cup	74	0
Teriyaki, bottled	¼ cup	60	0
Tomato, canned	1 cup	74	0.4
Worcestershire, bottled	1 tsp	0	0

Saturated Fat (g)	% Calories from Fat	% Calories from Saturated Fat	Cholesterol (mg)
0	17.7	0	0
0.1	2	<1	0
0	1.1	<1	0
0	3.3	<1	0
0.2	48	6	0
0.1	9	4.5	0
0.1	9	9	0
0.2	18.9	9.5	1
0.7	40.6	20.3	2
0.8	65.1	15.3	1
0.4	39	12	1
0.2	21.1	3.8	0
0.6	44.5	6.4	0
0	8.2	<1	0
0.9	39.4	6	0
0	<1	0	0
0	0	0	0
0.1	4.9	1.2	0
0	0	0	0

(continued)

Food	Portion	Calories	Fat (g)
Gravies and Sauces *(cont.)*			
Sauces *(cont.)*			
HIGH			
Alfredo, canned	½ cup	310	27
Bernaise, dry mix, made with milk and butter	¼ cup	175	17.1
Curry, dry mix, made with milk	¼ cup	67	3.7
Hollandaise, dry mix, made with milk and butter	¼ cup	176	17.1
Tartar	1 Tbsp	74	8.1
White			
dry mix, made with milk	¼ cup	60	3.4
medium, homemade	¼ cup	101	7.8
Ice Cream and Frozen Treats			
LOW			
Frozen yogurt, vanilla, fat-free	½ cup	110	0
Fruit ice	1 cup	247	0
Fruit juice bar	1 (about 1¾ oz)	42	0
ACCEPTABLE			
Frozen yogurt, vanilla	½ cup	110	1.5
Ice cream, vanilla, low-fat	½ cup	100	2
Sherbet, orange	½ cup	135	1.9
Tofutti, all flavors	½ cup	217	12
HIGH			
Frozen yogurt, cherry, premium	½ cup	110	2.5
Ice cream, soft-serve, chocolate or vanilla, on cone	1 (about 5 oz)	230	7
Ice cream, vanilla			
reduced-fat	½ cup	130	4.5
regular	½ cup	170	10
Ice cream sundae, chocolate	1 (about 6 oz)	300	7
Ice milk, soft-serve, vanilla	½ cup	112	2.3

Saturated Fat (g)	% Calories from Fat	% Calories from Saturated Fat	Cholesterol (mg)
15	78.4	43.5	75
10.5	87.9	54	47
1.5	49.7	20.1	9
10.5	87.4	53.7	47
1.5	98.5	18.4	7
1.6	51	24	9
4.3	69.5	38.3	26
0	0	0	0
0	0	0	0
0	0	0	0
1	12.3	8.2	5
1	18	9	5
1.2	12.7	8	7
2	49.8	8.3	0
1.5	20.5	12.3	10
5	27.4	19.6	20
3	31.2	20.8	35
6	52.9	31.8	105
5	21	15	20
1.4	18.5	11.3	7

(continued)

Food	Portion	Calories	Fat (g)
Meats			
Beef			
ACCEPTABLE			
Steak, top round, lean, broiled	3 oz	153	4.2
HIGH			
Brisket, lean, braised	3 oz	206	10.9
Corned beef hash, canned	1 cup	398	24.9
Ground, broiled			
extra-lean	3 oz	225	13.4
lean	3 oz	238	15
regular	3 oz	248	16.5
Liver, braised	3 oz	137	4.2
Meat loaf	3 oz	170	11.2
Roast			
bottom round, lean, braised	3 oz	178	7
pot, arm, lean, braised	3 oz	184	7.1
Shank cross cut, lean, simmered	3 oz	171	5.4
Short rib, lean, braised	3 oz	251	15.4
Steak			
filet mignon, lean, broiled	3 oz	179	8.5
flank, lean, broiled	3 oz	176	8.6
porterhouse, lean, broiled	3 oz	185	9.2
rib eye, lean, broiled	3 oz	191	10
sirloin, wedge bone, lean, broiled	3 oz	166	6.1
T-bone, lean, broiled	3 oz	182	8.8
Lamb			
HIGH			
Ground, broiled	3 oz	241	16.7
Kebab cubes, lean, broiled	3 oz	156	6.2
Leg, lean, roasted	3 oz	162	6.6
Rib roast, crown, lean, roasted	3 oz	197	11.3

Saturated Fat (g)	% Calories from Fat	% Calories from Saturated Fat	Cholesterol (mg)
1.4	24.7	8.2	71
3.9	47.6	17	79
11.9	56.3	26.9	73
5.3	53.6	21.2	84
5.9	56.7	22.3	86
6.5	59.9	23.6	86
1.6	27.6	10.5	331
5.1	59.3	27	55
2.4	35.4	12.1	82
2.6	34.7	12.7	86
2	28.4	10.5	66
6.6	55.2	23.7	79
3.2	42.7	16.1	71
3.7	44	18.9	57
3.7	44.8	18	68
4	47.1	18.8	68
2.4	33.1	13	76
3.5	43.5	17.3	68
6.9	62.4	25.8	82
2.2	35.8	12.7	77
2.4	36.7	13.3	76
4.1	51.6	18.7	75

(continued)

Food	Portion	Calories	Fat (g)
Meats *(cont.)*			
Lunchmeats/Processed Meats			
LOW			
Turkey breast	2 slices (about 1½ oz total)	47	0.7
HIGH			
Bologna			
beef	2 slices (about 2 oz total)	177	16.2
turkey	2 slices (about 2 oz total)	113	8.6
Chicken roll, light meat	2 slices (about 2 oz total)	90	4.2
Corned beef	2 slices (about 2 oz total)	142	8.5
Frankfurter			
beef	1	180	16.3
chicken	1	116	8.8
Ham, boiled, extra-lean	2 slices (about 2 oz total)	74	2.8
Liverwurst, fresh	3 slices (about 2 oz total)	185	16.2
Olive loaf	2 slices (about 2 oz total)	133	9.4
Pastrami			
beef	2 slices (about 2 oz total)	198	16.6
turkey	2 slices (about 2 oz total)	80	3.5
Pepperoni	10 slices (about 2 oz total)	273	24.2
Salami, pork	3 slices (about 2 oz total)	230	19.1

Saturated Fat (g)	% Calories from Fat	% Calories from Saturated Fat	Cholesterol (mg)
0.2	13.4	3.8	17
6.9	82.4	35.1	33
2.9	68.5	23.1	56
1.2	42	12	28
3.5	53.9	22.2	49
6.9	81.5	34.5	35
2.5	68.3	19.4	45
0.9	34.1	10.9	27
6	78.8	29.2	90
3.3	63.6	22.3	22
5.9	75.5	26.8	53
1	39.4	11.3	31
8.9	79.8	29.3	44
6.7	74.7	26.2	45

(continued)

Food	Portion	Calories	Fat (g)
Meats *(cont.)*			
Lunchmeats/Processed Meats *(cont.)*			
HIGH *(cont.)*			
Sausage			
bratwurst, fresh	1 link (about 3 oz)	256	22
kielbasa, smoked	2 slices (about 2 oz total)	176	15.4
knockwurst, smoked	1 link (about 2½ oz)	209	18.9
pork, fresh	4 links (about 2 oz total)	192	16.2
scrapple	2 oz	120	7.6
Turkey ham	2 slices (about 2 oz total)	73	2.8
Pork			
HIGH			
Bacon			
Canadian	2 medium slices (about 1½ oz total)	86	3.9
smoked	3 medium slices (about ¾ oz total)	109	9.4
smoked, thickly sliced	1 slice (about ⅓ oz)	50	4.5
Chop, center rib, lean, roasted	3 oz	208	11.7
Ham, cured, roasted	3 oz	140	6.5
Roast, center loin, lean, roasted	3 oz	204	11.1
Spareribs, lean, braised	3 oz	337	25.8
Veal			
HIGH			
Ground, broiled	3 oz	146	6.4
Loin, lean, roasted	3 oz	149	5.9

Saturated Fat (g)	% Calories from Fat	% Calories from Saturated Fat	Cholesterol (mg)
7.9	77.3	27.8	51
5.6	78.8	28.6	38
6.9	81.4	29.7	39
5.6	75.9	26.3	43
2.8	57	21	25
1	34.5	12.3	32
1.3	40.8	13.6	27
3.3	77.6	27.2	16
2	81	36	10
4.1	50.6	17.7	67
2.2	41.8	14.1	48
3.8	49	16.8	77
10	68.9	26.7	103
2.6	39.5	16	88
2.2	35.6	13.3	90

(continued)

Food	Portion	Calories	Fat (g)
Milk and Milk Products			
Cream			
LOW			
Sour cream, fat-free	2 Tbsp	30	0
HIGH			
Half-and-half	2 Tbsp	39	3.5
Heavy	2 Tbsp	103	11
Light	2 Tbsp	59	5.8
Nondairy, powdered	1 tsp	10	0.5
flavored	1 tsp	60	3
Sour cream			
reduced-fat	2 Tbsp	35	2
regular	2 Tbsp	62	6
Whipped cream	2 Tbsp	19	1.7
Whipped topping, nondairy	2 Tbsp	30	2.4
Milk			
LOW			
Dairy shake mix, chocolate, prepared with water	About 6 oz	80	1
Dry, nonfat, prepared	1 cup	82	0.2
Evaporated, fat-free	2 Tbsp	25	0
Fat-free	1 cup	86	0.4
ACCEPTABLE			
1% low-fat, chocolate	1 cup	158	2.5
HIGH			
Buttermilk	1 cup	99	2.2
Eggnog	½ cup	171	9.5
Evaporated	2 Tbsp	40	2
1%	1 cup	102	2.6
2%	1 cup	121	4.7

Saturated Fat (g)	% Calories from Fat	% Calories from Saturated Fat	Cholesterol (mg)
0	0	0	2
2.2	80.8	50.8	11
6.9	96.1	60.3	41
3.6	88.5	54.9	20
0.5	45	45	0
2.5	45	37.5	0
1.5	51.4	38.6	10
3.8	87.1	55.2	13
1	80.5	47.4	6
2	72	60	0
0	11.3	0	0
0.1	2.2	1.1	4
0	0	0	0
0.3	4.2	3.1	4
1.5	14.2	8.5	7
1.3	20	11.8	9
5.7	50	30	75
1	45	22.5	5
1.6	22.9	14.1	10
2.9	35	21.6	18

(continued)

Food	Portion	Calories	Fat (g)
Milk (cont.)			
Milk and Milk Products (cont.)			
HIGH (cont.)			
Whole	1 cup	157	8.9
Whole, chocolate	1 cup	208	8.5
Yogurt			
LOW			
Fruit			
light (low-calorie)	1 cup	100	0
regular	1 cup	240	3
Fruit with crunch-type topping			
light (low-calorie)	$^3/_4$ cup	130	1
regular	$^3/_4$ cup	220	2
Plain, fat-free	1 cup	120	0
HIGH			
Plain			
low-fat (1$^1/_2$% milk fat)	1 cup	150	4
whole milk	1 cup	139	7.4
Nuts and Seeds			
Nuts			
LOW			
Chestnuts, European, roasted	1 oz	70	0.6
Filberts (hazelnuts), unblanched, dried	1 oz	179	17.8
ACCEPTABLE			
Almonds, unblanched, dried	1 oz	167	14.8
Pecans, dried	1 oz	189	19.2
Pistachios, dried	1 oz	164	13.7
Walnuts, English, dried	1 oz	182	17.6
HIGH			
Brazil, unblanched, dried	1 oz	186	18.8
Cashews, dry-roasted	1 oz	163	13.2

Saturated Fat (g)	% Calories from Fat	% Calories from Saturated Fat	Cholesterol (mg)
5.6	51	32.1	35
5.3	36.8	22.9	31
0	0	0	0
1.5	11.3	5.6	15
0	6.9	0	0
0.5	8.2	2	<5
0	0	0	0
2.5	24	15	20
4.8	47.9	31.1	29
0.1	7.7	1.3	0
1.3	89.5	6.5	0
1.4	79.8	7.5	0
1.5	91.4	7.1	0
1.7	75.2	9.3	0
1.6	87	7.9	0
4.6	91	22.3	0
2.6	72.9	14.4	0

(continued)

Food	Portion	Calories	Fat (g)
Nuts and Seeds *(cont.)*			
Nuts			
HIGH *(cont.)*			
Coconut, sweetened, flaked	1 oz	126	9
Macadamia, dried	1 oz	199	20.9
Mixed, dry-roasted	1 oz	169	14.6
Peanuts, dry-roasted	1 oz	164	13.9
Pine, pignolia, dried	1 oz	146	14.4
Seeds			
ACCEPTABLE			
Sunflower, dried	1 oz	162	14.1
HIGH			
Pumpkin, dried, hulled	1 oz	154	13
Sesame, dried, hulled	1 Tbsp	47	4.4
Pasta			
LOW			
Fresh, cooked	1 cup	183	1.5
Macaroni, enriched, cooked	1 cup	197	0.9
Noodles			
egg, enriched, cooked	1 cup	213	2.4
soba, cooked	1 cup	113	0.1
spinach, enriched, cooked	1 cup	211	2.5
Spaghetti			
enriched, cooked	1 cup	197	0.9
whole wheat, cooked	1 cup	174	0.8
Spinach, fresh, cooked	1 cup	182	1.3
Vegetable, cooked	³⁄₄ cup	210	1
HIGH			
Tortellini, cheese	¹⁄₂ cup	220	5

Saturated Fat (g)	% Calories from Fat	% Calories from Saturated Fat	Cholesterol (mg)
8	64.3	57.1	0
3.1	94.5	14	0
2	77.8	10.7	0
1.9	76.3	10.4	0
2.2	88.8	13.6	0
1.5	78.3	8.3	0
2.5	76	14.6	0
0.6	84.3	11.5	0
0.2	7.4	1	46
0.1	4.1	<1	0
0.5	10.1	2.1	53
0	<1	<1	0
0.6	10.7	2.6	53
0.1	4.1	<1	0
0.1	4.1	<1	0
0.3	6.4	1.5	46
0	4.3	0	0
3	20.5	12.3	40

(continued)

Food	Portion	Calories	Fat (g)
Pasta Dishes			
LOW			
Pasta salad with seafood, without dressing	3½ oz	90	5
ACCEPTABLE			
Lasagna with meat sauce, low-fat, frozen	About 10 oz	312	6.9
Pasta primavera, frozen	About 10 oz	260	8
Spaghetti and meatballs, homemade	1 cup	332	11.7
HIGH			
Fettuccine Alfredo, frozen	About 9 oz	270	7
Lasagna with meat sauce, frozen	About 10 oz	377	14
Macaroni and cheese, homemade, baked	1 cup	430	22.2
Manicotti, cheese, frozen	About 3 oz	290	9
Ravioli, cheese, with tomato sauce, frozen	About 9½ oz	360	14
Tortellini, cheese, with tomato sauce, frozen	About 9 oz	290	6
Pizza			
LOW			
Cheese			
Healthy Choice French bread pizza	1 (about 5½ oz)	310	4
Italian sausage			
Healthy Choice sausage French bread pizza	1 (about 6 oz)	330	4
Supreme Lean Cuisine deluxe French bread pizza	1 (about 6 oz)	330	6
ACCEPTABLE			
Cheese			
Chef Boyardee, dry mix, prepared	1 slice (about 5 oz)	320	8
Weight Watchers extra cheese	1 (about 5¾ oz)	390	12

Saturated Fat (g)	% Calories from Fat	% Calories from Saturated Fat	Cholesterol (mg)
0.6	50	6	12
3	19.8	8.6	22
2.5	27.7	8.7	35
3.3	31.7	8.9	74
3	23.3	10	15
2.2	33.5	15.9	45
8.9	46.5	18.6	42
3.5	27.9	10.9	20
5	35	12.5	85
5	18.6	15.5	105
2	11.6	5.8	10
1.5	10.9	4.1	20
2.5	16.4	6.8	30
2.5	22.5	7	15
4	27.7	9.2	35

(continued)

Food	Portion	Calories	Fat (g)
Pizza (cont.)			
ACCEPTABLE (cont.)			
Pepperoni			
Weight Watchers	1 (about 5½ oz)	390	12
Supreme			
Weight Watchers deluxe combo	1 (about 6½ oz)	380	11
HIGH			
Cheese			
Domino's thin crust	⅓ of 12″ pie (about 5½ oz)	364	15.5
Pizza Hut thin crust	1 slice of medium pie (about 3½ oz)	205	8
Italian sausage			
Domino's hand-tossed, with mushrooms	2 slices of 12″ pie (about 6 oz)	402	13.9
Pizza Hut hand-tossed	1 slice of medium pie (about 4 oz)	267	11
Pepperoni			
Domino's hand-tossed	2 slices of 12″ pie (about 6 oz)	406	15.1
Healthy Choice pepperoni French bread pizza	1 (about 6 oz)	350	9
Pizza Hut hand-tossed	1 slice of medium pie (about 4 oz)	238	8
Supreme			
Pizza Hut hand-tossed	1 slice of medium pie (about 5 oz)	284	12
Veggie			
Domino's hand-tossed	2 slices of 12″ pie (about 6¾ oz total)	360	10.4
Pizza Hut hand-tossed	1 slice of medium pie (about 5 oz)	216	6
Poultry, Fowl, and Game			
LOW			
Chicken breast, without skin			
fried in batter	½ (about 3 oz)	161	4.1
roasted	½ (about 3 oz)	142	3.1

Saturated Fat (g)	% Calories from Fat	% Calories from Saturated Fat	Cholesterol (mg)
4	27.7	9.2	45
3.5	26.1	8.3	40
6.3	38.3	15.6	26
4	35.1	17.6	25
6.1	31.1	13.7	31
5	37	16	31
6.6	33.8	14.6	32
4	23.1	10.3	25
4	30.3	15.1	24
5	38	15.8	30
4.5	26	11.3	19
3	25	12.5	17
1.1	22.9	6.1	78
0.9	19.6	5.7	73

(continued)

Food	Portion	Calories	Fat (g)
Poultry, Fowl, and Game *(cont.)*			
LOW *(cont.)*			
Frogs' legs, uncooked	3 oz	62	0.3
Turkey			
breast, prebasted, roasted, without skin	3 oz	107	2.9
light meat, roasted, without skin	3 oz	34	0.7
ACCEPTABLE			
Pheasant, meat only, uncooked	3 oz	113	3.1
Venison, roasted	3 oz	134	2.7
HIGH			
Capon, roasted, without skin	3 oz	195	9.9
Chicken			
breast, with skin			
fried in batter	$\frac{1}{2}$ (about 5 oz)	364	18.5
roasted	$\frac{1}{2}$ (about 4 oz)	193	7.6
roasted, ready-to-serve	$\frac{1}{2}$ (about 5 oz)	250	13
drumstick, with skin			
fried in batter	1 (about 3 oz)	193	11.3
roasted	1 (about 2 oz)	112	5.8
liver, simmered	3 oz	133	4.6
thigh, without skin			
fried in batter	1 (about 2 oz)	113	5.4
roasted	1 (about 2 oz)	109	5.7
Duck, roasted, without skin	3 oz	171	9.5
Pâté			
chicken, canned	1 oz	57	3.7
goose, smoked, canned	1 oz	131	12.4
Potpie, turkey, homemade	1 piece (about 8 oz)	550	31.3
Rabbit, roasted	3 oz	131	5.4
Squab (pigeon), uncooked	1 (about 6 oz)	239	12.6

Saturated Fat (g)	% Calories from Fat	% Calories from Saturated Fat	Cholesterol (mg)
0	4.4	0	43
0.8	24.4	6.7	36
0.2	18.5	5.3	15
1.1	24.7	8.8	56
1.1	18.1	7.4	95
2.8	45.7	12.9	73
4.9	45.7	12.1	119
2.2	35.4	10.3	82
4	46.8	14.4	110
3	52.7	14	62
1.6	46.6	12.9	47
1.6	31.1	10.8	536
1.5	43	11.9	53
1.6	47.1	13.2	49
3.6	50	18.9	76
1.1	58.4	17.4	111
4.1	85.2	28.2	43
10.5	51.2	17.2	72
1.6	37.1	11	54
3.3	47.4	12.4	151

(continued)

Food	Portion	Calories	Fat (g)
Poultry, Fowl, and Game *(cont.)*			
HIGH *(cont.)*			
Turkey			
dark meat, roasted, without skin	3 oz	32	1.2
dark meat, roasted, with skin	3 oz	188	9.8
light meat, roasted, with skin	3 oz	168	7.1
liver, simmered	3 oz	144	5.1
Soups and Stews			
Soups			
LOW			
Black bean, condensed, made with water	1 cup	116	1.5
Clam chowder			
Manhattan, condensed, made with water	1 cup	78	2.2
New England, low-fat	1 cup	120	2
Crab	1 cup	76	1.5
Gazpacho	1 cup	56	2.2
Minestrone, low-fat	1 cup	120	2
Onion, condensed, made with water	1 cup	58	1.7
Split pea with ham, low-fat	1 cup	170	2.5
Tomato			
condensed, made with water	½ cup	100	2
low-fat	½ cup	90	2
Vegetarian vegetable, condensed, made with water	1 cup	72	1.9
ACCEPTABLE			
Bouillon, chicken, from cube, made with water	1 cup	12	0.3
Chicken noodle, condensed, made with water	1 cup	75	2.5
Chicken rice, condensed, made with water	1 cup	60	1.9
Green pea, condensed, made with water	1 cup	165	2.9
Lentil with ham	1 cup	139	2.8

Saturated Fat (g)	% Calories from Fat	% Calories from Saturated Fat	Cholesterol (mg)
0.4	33.8	11.3	15
3	46.9	14.4	76
2	38	10.7	65
1.6	31.9	10	532
0.4	11.6	3.1	0
0.4	25.4	4.6	2
0.5	15	3.8	5
0.4	17.8	4.7	10
0.3	35.4	4.8	0
0.5	15	3.8	<1
0.3	26.4	4.7	0
1	13.2	5.3	10
0	18	0	0
0.5	20	5	0
0.3	23.8	3.8	0
0.1	22.5	7.5	0
0.7	30	8.4	7
0.5	28.5	7.5	7
1.4	15.8	7.6	0
1.1	18.1	7.1	7

(continued)

Food	Portion	Calories	Fat (g)
Soups and Stews (cont.)			
Soups (cont.)			
HIGH			
Beef noodle, condensed, made with water	1 cup	83	3.1
Beef vegetable, condensed, made with water	1 cup	78	1.9
Bouillon, beef, from cube, made with water	1 cup	7	0.2
Cheese, condensed, made with water	1 cup	156	10.5
Cream of celery, condensed, made with water	1 cup	90	5.6
Cream of chicken, condensed, made with water	1 cup	117	7.4
Cream of mushroom, condensed, made with water	1 cup	129	9
Cream of potato, condensed, made with water	1 cup	73	2.4
Scotch broth, condensed, made with water	1 cup	80	2.6
Turkey vegetable, condensed, made with water	1 cup	72	3
Stews			
HIGH			
Beef, ready-to-serve	1 cup	194	7.6
Oyster, condensed, made with water	1 cup	58	3.8
Vegetables			
LOW			
Broccoli, boiled	½ cup	22	0.3
Cabbage, boiled, shredded	½ cup	17	0.3
Carrot, raw	1 (about 7½", 2½ oz)	31	0.1
Chile peppers, raw, chopped	½ cup	30	0.2
Corn, sweet yellow, boiled	Kernels from 1 ear	83	1
Eggplant, boiled, cubed	½ cup	13	0.1

Saturated Fat (g)	% Calories from Fat	% Calories from Saturated Fat	Cholesterol (mg)
1.2	33.6	13	5
0.9	21.9	10.4	5
0.1	25.7	12.9	0
6.7	60.6	38.7	30
1.4	56	14	15
2.1	56.9	16.2	10
2.4	62.8	16.7	2
1.2	29.6	14.8	5
1.1	29.3	12.4	5
0.9	37.5	11.3	2
2.5	35.3	11.6	34
2.5	59	38.8	14
0	12.3	1.6	0
0	15.9	2.1	0
0	2.9	<1	0
0	6	<1	0
0.2	10.8	2.2	0
0	6.9	1.4	0

(continued)

Food	Portion	Calories	Fat (g)
Vegetables *(cont.)*			
LOW *(cont.)*			
Garlic, raw	1 clove	4	0
Okra, boiled	½ cup	26	0.1
Onions, raw, chopped	½ cup	30	0.1
Pumpkin, canned	½ cup	41	0.3
Tomatoes, raw, chopped	1 cup	38	0.6
Zucchini, raw, sliced	½ cup	9	0.1
Potatoes			
LOW			
Baked			
plain, flesh only	1 (about 6 oz)	145	0.2
plain, microwaved, flesh and skin	1 (about 8 oz)	212	0.2
Boiled, flesh only	1	67	0.1
Sweet potato, baked	1 (about 4 oz)	117	0.1
ACCEPTABLE			
Mashed, made with whole milk and margarine	½ cup	111	4.4
O'Brien	½ cup	79	1.2
Potato salad	½ cup	179	10.3
HIGH			
Au gratin	½ cup	161	9.2
Baked, with sour cream and chives	1 (about 6 oz)	221	12.6
French fries			
deep-fried	20–25 1"–2" strips	235	12.2
frozen, oven-heated	20 (about 4 oz total)	222	8.8
microwave	1 box (about 3 oz)	230	12
Potato pancake	1 (about 3 oz)	234	12.6
Scalloped	½ cup	105	4.5

Saturated Fat (g)	% Calories from Fat	% Calories from Saturated Fat	Cholesterol (mg)
0	4.5	0	0
0	3.5	1.4	0
0	3	<1	0
0.2	6.6	4.4	0
0.1	14.2	2.4	0
0	10	2	0
0	1.2	<1	0
0.1	<1	<1	0
0	1.3	<1	0
0	<1	<1	0
1.1	35.7	8.9	2
0.8	13.7	9.1	4
1.8	51.8	9.1	85
5.8	51.4	32.4	28
5.6	51.3	22.8	14
3.8	46.7	14.6	0
4.5	35.7	18.2	0
3	47	11.7	0
3.4	48.5	13.1	93
2.8	38.6	24	15

Y

Z